Mastering Your Masculinity

How to Become Good at Being a Man

KEN CURRY, LMFT

DEDICATION

This one is for Paul Denman Curry, my Dad.

CONTENTS

ACKNOWLEDGMENTS

Thanks to my family who has been alongside me as I have developed this process. You have seen my struggles and personal development in real time right in front of you. Your feedback and support has been so important to me.

Thanks to the men of my groups. Your courage and ability to rise to all the challenges that I have given you will always be an inspiration. You have been the benefactors of this process and my appreciation goes to you for being the "guinea pigs" as this process was discovered and developed.

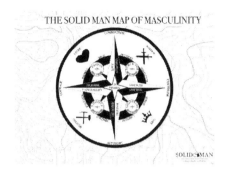

1 Introduction

Welcome to the Solid Man Process. Presently our world is experiencing a significant loss. Something vital is missing for the health and structure of our world. Even though you may not recognize what it is, you have felt this loss on a personal level. It's probably why you're reading this.

For decades now, what we believe about men and the role of men in family and society has been questioned. While initially this scrutiny was necessary because some things needed to be questioned, it has resulted in enormous changes in the narrative about what we believe about the value and worth of men. Because of this, you may have wondered about your own value or questioned whether it is even good to be a man.

How men interact with and influence the world has been under the microscope. The result has been confusion and uncertainty about the role of men. Because of this turmoil, many men have lost (or discarded) the good, strong core of their manhood.

The Solid Man Process is designed to help men reclaim that center, so the entire world can experience good, positive Masculinity.

Usually men's "work" tries to fix what's wrong with you. With this process, we will release what is right about you. Some men think something in our essence is our enemy that needs to be reined in. So, we fight ourselves as though we are our own enemy. In this process, we will let go of that fight, eliminating self-attack and listening to the real challenges that being a man presents to us every day.

This process will uncover a deeper framework within you and help you develop a set of skills and practices designed for change. It is a holistic approach which respects the integration of body, heart, spirit and community. The Solid Man process establishes the foundation that nothing is wrong with you, you are in good working order and you have a tremendous amount of Internal Resources on hand.

The Solid Man Process is about empowering every man. The more a man becomes personally empowered the more likely he will reach his potential and make a powerful and positive impact on the world.

What goes on in a man's heart, mind and spirit has a powerful influence on all aspects of life. When he becomes who he is meant to be, his life begins to become the greatest version of what it was meant to be.

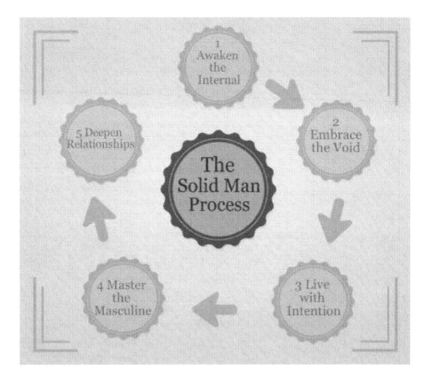

This journey is most effective when done with other men. Invite and gather a few men to go through this journey with you. Since this is a lifetime process, you'll need to be ready to learn, listen and interact with other men.

Review of Pillar One

The first book (Pillar One) in this series, *Awakening the Internal*, was designed to help you develop an internally referenced life to become awake, strong, and alive in your life. This is essential work in order for you to live in freedom and mastery in your life.

Pillar One outlined the problem that we are and have been externally referenced. *Awakening the Internal* challenged you to shift from being externally defined and driven to being internally defined and driven. If there is one thing that we need to continue building strength, it is to become internally defined and driven!

This is the most significant shift a man must make in his life to become a Solid Man, to develop an internal identity and internal motivation in your life so that you live out who you really are. You will never become fully free until you are able to unplug from the motherboard of externals. External validation has been our drug of choice – you've been smoking the validation crackpipe! This must change.

As you move toward freedom in your life you will experience more peace and have a more settled or centered life experience. Your journey has been to develop a solid core of integrity and to develop an integrated life, pulling all the categories of your internal life together in good working order.

You've made some significant gains in your life, relationships, work and family. It is imperative to keep this going. You must continue to be aware, conscious and observe what is going on internally and around you. Your emotions, intuition, body, spirit and mind will lead you well.

You will do just fine if you listen to yourself and trust your internal processes. You have all the tools within you to live a solid life. Remember where you've come from, all the steps you've made and where you want to be. You can do this!

Review of Pillar Two

Pillar Two is called *Embracing the Void*. It is the second book in the Solid Man process that helps you to get your heart back, along with building your courage and confidence. You learned how to engage in a part of life that most people avoid like the plague, the Void. You found that embracing the Void is the pathway to being initiated toward becoming a man.

Pillar Two challenged you to Embrace the Void. We outlined what the Void is and how it has been designed to bring about growth, maturity and strength in your life. The Void is the pathway into the sacred and holy aspects of life that can only be experienced if we intentionally enter into our Void experiences.

We learned that most of us do everything we can to avoid the Void, using many different avenues of avoidance like addictions, control, and passivity. We learned that the Void is a normal and vital part of human existence. Our initiation into manhood is brought about by facing and engaging with the uncertainty of the Void. The Void creates competent and confident men.

Review of Pillar Three

Living With Intention is Pillar Three and is about building a core of integrity. We all struggle with the same core issue, even if the symptoms are different on the outside; lack of a solid core.

Having a strong internal sense of integrity is essential to becoming the man you want to be and creating the life you want.

In Pillar Three helped you answer five significant Core questions so you could move with intention and purpose in your life. Most men live with an externally referenced motivation and drive. The work of Pillar Three opened up your awareness to deeper inner realities to assist you in becoming more intentionally referenced with your internal core.

The journey of Pillar Three moved you deeply into more Solid Manhood. You discovered five movements into deeper connection with Source and Self. Each of these movements has one question to be answered and one practice in which to become proficient.

Where does life come from?   Anchoring

Who am I?   Remembering

What do I need?   Self-care

What do I want?   Living from your heart

Where am I going?   Creating

4

Overview of Pillar Four

Pillar Four will explore the often-mysterious concept of Masculinity. We will look into how to take what you have learned thus far and apply the internally referenced life toward becoming good at being a man. You will learn how to Master your Masculinity.

The purpose of Pillar Four is to create a map that will outline some significant aspects of manhood and Masculinity. Within the cultural context in which we now find ourselves, there are many opinions, expectations and representations of what Masculinity is or ought to be.

The Solid Man Process is designed to set men free to be who they are as individuals, to make a positive impact on the world around them and to give each man a solid sense of identity and integrity.

Pillar Four will break through some of the confusion that men have been experiencing as they walk through life. I provide a clear path.

This Pillar is about becoming a good man and becoming good at being a man.

Being a good man is about being the best masculine human being you possibly could be. It is taking all the tools you have been given, developing wisdom and doing the right thing as often as possible. It is about keeping your own personal house in order so that you can thrive while also having a positive influence on the world around you.

Becoming good at being a man is about understanding the depth and calling of your Masculinity and manhood. You will develop a clear understanding of what Masculinity is, what it is designed for and then begin practicing building proficiency, even mastery, as you move through life as a masculine being.

From the previous Pillars you know you have the goods and the internal tools to master life and relationships already within you. Here, we will take all those tools and incorporate with one of the most profound internal realities, your Masculinity.

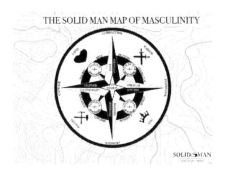

THE SOLID MAN MAP OF MASCULINITY

SOLID MAN

2 What Is Masculinity?

Factors of Masculinity

For some reason you have this book in your hands because you want to thrive, be the best man you can be and get the most out of life. We all are on a journey through life, some to just survive or get by, some to thrive.

This book is for men who want to master their Masculinity. There are many views on what Masculinity is, and I am throwing my ideas into the conversation. This is for men who see themselves as men, who want to be men and who want to become the best man they can be. It doesn't matter if you are Christian or atheist, from whatever cultural heritage or even straight or gay, this is for men who want to master being good at being a man.

I am an observant person watching what is unfolding in our culture today, I come from a fairly old-school mind-set, I am a Christian man and I have my opinions (as you will see), but the most important opinion as you begin reading this is that your life is best lived from an internal rather than external reference, that is your opinion. I taught this in Pillar One, but it needs reinforcing. Building your internal frame is essential to live with integrity. You have powerful internal resources that guide every moment of your life in real time. One of your most profound internal resources is your Masculinity.

As men who are building an internal frame of reference, your challenge as you read this is to consider how you will build Masculinity the way you want to build it. It is your choice how to build every concept into your life as you see fit. I will be laying out a significant framework, a map which will outline important characteristics of manhood, your job is to take those concepts and make them your own.

I will show you a map, but the map is not the territory. The territory is you. Where all this interacts with the world, with real relationships and in real time is in your body, heart and soul, in you. You are the real deal, so make it so.

This book is an exploration to answer the question, "What is Masculinity?" First, I will give a lay of the land with some concepts which describe where we are as a country with the discussion about manhood. I'll lay out some other thoughts I have and then we will jump into what I believe are the central aspects that are essential to Masculinity and how it is best developed. Let's start with the context in which we find ourselves having this conversation.

Idea or Fact

The degree to which you believe Masculinity is an idea constructed through cultural agreements and interactions or if it is a "brute" fact that exists apart from culture or language will determine the foundation upon which you will build your perception of Masculinity as a personal internal or external reality.

An "idea" is a concept that has been developed over time within a certain culture and now has been defined with certain characteristics and value. The idea could be something like the presidency of the United States, an academic institution or a dollar bill. As an idea, the dollar is just a piece of paper backed up by a promise that it actually has value. An idea is a concept, not necessarily a reality.

An example of a brute fact would be gravity; gravity is gravity in any language or even in no language, it simply is what it is. The same is with the ocean, breathing or anything else that just "is". No matter what it is, it still has substance, a construct and essence; it does not matter what it is called, how it is described or even who describes it, it is what it is and does what it does.

Think of these concepts as a spectrum, with nurture on one side and nature on the other. One side of the spectrum that is nurture is the side of those who believe Masculinity is a culturally constructed idea, not a hard fact. As well, those who believe this are loathe to consider any idea of Masculinity that transcends any of the various cultures in our world. It is though each culture has developed their certain "idea" or version of Masculinity unique to that culture.

Idea ———————————————————— Fact

Considering Masculinity as an "idea" places Masculinity in the position of being an "ought". Masculinity "ought" to be this way or that way depending on any one perception. "Ought" thinking opens the discussion to any and every concept of what a man who is masculine may or may not be. Therefore, anyone with influence can potentially determine not just what Masculinity is but can also determine its value.

> ☞ **If Masculinity is an "ought", anyone can define it.**

The cultural trends that exist at that particular moment in history are able to designate how and why the masculine is expressed as acceptable or not. At that point, present fads or pop culture determine the value of the masculine.

Many who profess the idea, nurture or culture side of the spectrum, believe in the concept of *Tabula Rasa*, which means that every human being is born with no on-board or inherent gender. You are a blank slate upon which your parents and culture determine how you move and exist with whatever gender they decide you will have.

In this line of thinking, most everything with how Masculinity is lived out or how Masculinity is defined by how people taught what was acceptable behavior, how a man or boy was supposed to act or be.

Generally, this is the worldview of many social constructionists, social justice warriors, and academics. This mindset usually is centered around externals that have to do with behaviors and "do's". Often, they will use lists called "man rules" which are often just a list of random external expectations of what they think men think another man is; such as a "real" man has sex with many women, never shows emotion or always wins.

> ☞ **The Man Rules are just external expectations.**

These generated lists of external behaviors are used to show the reality of how men really are, but usually just reveal how inept people think men are in life, in relationship or some other negative view. These stereotypes and lists of rules never actually speak reality to what is or even what ought to be, just what is envisioned as an idea in someone's mind designed to shift behavior toward what is socially acceptable to this group. It's a kind of social engineering using shame and misandry to compel men to behave "properly" and not in a "toxic" fashion.

In August 2018, the American Psychological Association (APA) came out with guidelines for therapy with boys and men.

Here's the first guideline; "Psychologists strive to recognize that masculinities are constructed based on social, cultural, and contextual norms." This sets forth a very clear opinion upon which the APA suggests or recommends as specific professional behavior, endeavor, or conduct for psychologists. They have announced very clearly upon which side of the equation they sit, they say that Masculinity is a social construction, an idea.

The APA suggests that "Traditionally Masculine Traits" like stoicism, aggression, competitiveness and dominance hinder a man from being a healthy human being.

That's why Masculinity is thought of as "toxic" because to them, these four traits are obviously really bad. However, these traits are just things any human can express in healthy or unhealthy ways, just like any other trait.

Being stoic is necessary when taking a test or doing surgery, but at a funeral, it would not be as fitting. Physical aggression is necessary when standing up against a bully or for justice, but not so much with a toddler. We have all seen that guy who is overly competitive, it's an unhealthy expression of his lack of identity, but pursuing victory in a sport or in business is very healthy.

Dominance is the same, you cannot escape the fact that humanity has dominance hierarchies, it is healthy to lead and influence. But it is unhealthy when someone takes the power they have and forces another to submit. By trying to shame these traits out of men the APA and other influences in our society are attempting to gain power over men by defining what is ok and not ok with a masculine person. This behavior by the APA just seems like the toxic, hegemonic or controlling behavior they so despise.

Whether the list of expectations is an old set of rules or a new set of rules, what you need to see is this; for some Masculinity is determined by an external set of rules built by people who see Masculinity as an "idea".

Even though they say it is undefined or even undefinable, ironically, this is where these folks then do their best to then determine the definition of Masculinity on their terms. They have given themselves the high position of creating the narrative of what Masculinity is or is not. Very clever.

Nurture	Nature
(Idea)	(Fact)

The other side of the spectrum is the idea that Masculinity is a "brute fact". That is, Masculinity is imbedded within men's biology and physical DNA or there is a significant imprint of something that determines Masculinity from a deep internal place with in a man's soul, whether it is from a spiritual or archetypal source or from neurologic firmware within.

Within this mindset is the belief that either Masculinity has been developed purposefully over eons for the advancement and survival of the species (evolutionists and evolutionary psychologists), the grand narrative of heroic myths embedded within men (Mytho-poetics like Robert Bly and Sam Keen and Archetypists like Carl Jung) or it is by design, as men were created by God, in his image (creationists or intelligent design).

> ➔ So God created man in His own image; in the image of God He created him; male and female He created them. Genesis 1:27

It is interesting to think that "masculine as nature" is one place that evolutionists and creationists are strange bedfellows! Whether it is intelligent design or genetic mutations over time it is nature, within a man, Kum-ba-yah.

Eastern Religions also seem to sit on this side of the spectrum. The concept of Yin and Yang indicates that there is a polarity between the masculine and the feminine. They exist in two different energies, Yin with feminine and Yang with the masculine. There is a distinct energy with the masculine and with the feminine. I personally do not know much about this, except that Eastern religions notice this distinction between masculine and feminine.

As you do any reading or listening to any commentary on news or podcasts, consider what position that person is making with their ideas about men and Masculinity. Usually these two sides of the spectrum become obvious. These differences have created confusion, I want to reduce the confusion so that men can move forward with strength as masculine men.

> ➔ Masculinity is a deep internal construct within each man.

If you have read any Solid Man material, you can easily guess which side of the spectrum I rest; the nature side. I believe Masculinity is found in our nature, deep with the core of every man. As you read this material you will see there is also a strong aspect of nurture, this is done as other men take the natural, internal structure that exists within all men and "nurture" the masculine soul toward maturity.

Here's where I rest on this line. It is because other men must be involved by teaching and guiding young men and boys toward maturity. They will mentor the inherent internal structure toward its natural position of strength, confidence and presence.

Nurture	Solid Man	Nature
(Idea)		(Fact)

You may have heard of the so-called "crisis" in Masculinity. I don't believe there is any crisis with Masculinity, Masculinity is doing just fine. The crisis is in maturity, there just are not many good pathways toward mature Masculinity or good models of how to live out Masculinity in our present culture. We are in a world of confusion and lack of clarity.

It is true that men need to guide men into and toward strong, mature Masculinity, that is where nurture is required. We just don't have good avenues for that to happen much in our world today. Most men are kind of left to themselves to try to figure it out. The Solid Man work hopes to create new paths of good mentorship into strong, mature Masculinity.

> ⌕ **Young men need other men to guide them into mature Masculinity.**

The narrative that Masculinity is just an idea, and femininity or any gender for that matter is just a social construct, seems to be prevailing in the world of acadamia. Fortunately for most people, the academics influential reach is very limited. The "man on the street" just sees that he has masculine body parts and that common sense says something is just natural. When the academics say Masculinity is a concept made up by culture, our man somehow "knows" something else is true. Therefore, to him, this whole discussion we are having right now is an absurd waste of his time.

Consider what is out there; on one side we have the beta nice guy, the white knight or the SNAG (sensitive new-age guy); the Ray Romano's or Jerry Seinfeld's. These men have good hearts, but not much spine. On the other side we have the hyper-masculine alpha jerk that looks like any Swarzenegger or Stallone character; men with tons of spine, but not much heart.

There are a few models that show a good strong man with a beautiful measure of both heart and spine. You'll find many if you consider regular men in your world, there are many good men out there, men who are everyday heroes, hard workers, dads and men just doing their best to make life work.

● **Heart and Spine are two primary characteristics of Solid men.**

This book is called *Mastering Your Masculinity*, I'll show you primary components of what Masculinity looks like and then you'll make that happen with your own personality and internal character.

We don't have enough pathways present in our culture for developing good strong Masculinity. We have those who are pragmatically trying to find what works in life or the social constructionists who seem to have an agenda to influence culture in a certain direction.

Oddly, this pragmatism comes in the form of either the PUA (Pick Up Artist) world, trying to find what works to get a man laid, or the Christian world, what works to get men to be obedient to whatever the expectation of that particular tradition requires. These two have plenty to say about being a man, but sadly both usually miss the mark dramatically.

It is as though our society has become uncomfortable with masculine strength. It seems that there is a desire to remove Masculinity from the man while still mandating that they be strong. C. S. Lewis observed this long ago.

● "In a sort of ghastly simplicity, we remove the organ and demand the function. We make men without chests and expect of them virtue and enterprise. We laugh at honour and are shocked to find traitors in our midst. We castrate and bid the geldings be fruitful." — C.S. Lewis, The Abolition of Man

"We castrate and bid the geldings, be fruitful." Is a strong statement and it fits our world today like nothing I have ever read. The desire to remove Masculinity from men and then demand that they hold the same expectation is absurd and potentially evil.

The Solid Man Process is doing everything it can do to create good models and pathways for developing good solid masculine men. This is an endeavor to bring maturity back to the world of Masculinity.

Even if you lean over to the side that Masculinity is a social construct, I welcome you to join the journey of developing a strong, empowered masculine self. The Solid Man process is all about empowering each man to develop and master his own internally referenced person from his own internal resources. It doesn't matter where you think it all comes from, becoming the man <u>you</u> were meant to be, is our goal.

Masculinity is simply how a man interacts with the world. The world is a tough place to navigate, it is full of rules/limitations/boundaries and potential harm or death. Nature has brute realities that rule how you move through life. Those brute forces push against our being and at the same time are present within our being.

A masculine being moves with those forces as a masculine being would. A feminine being moves with those forces as a feminine person would. This is where the masculine or feminine is played out – in response to the brute world, which is what nature is.

However, it seems an underlying assumption in some worldviews exists that humans are above nature, that we have attained separation from the natural world through evolution or that we exist as beings that are inherently distanced from nature. I think this is why the concept of Masculinity as nature is a problem, or more precisely seeing humanity as part of nature is the problem.

From this perspective it might be said, "Since humanity is above the natural world and gender is part of that natural world, to be fully human a human must be separate from the natural world by removing any sense of masculine or feminine." Therefore, for those who hold this worldview, the next move as humans in the evolutionary process is the removal of all gender, masculine or feminine. This is especially true if the masculine and feminine are considered natural.

If humans were above or beyond nature, we would not be beholden to natural laws and humans would then be free to express themselves with whatever behavior is appealing at the time, there are no restrictions or limitations, you can do (or be) whatever you want and do whatever you please, but only if it fits with the "correct" trend of the moment. Here I am talking about breaking free from the restrictions of nature.

It would be absurd if it was breaking free from gravity. It is also a desire to break free from any spiritual restriction as well. It is the teenage cry, "I can do what I want!"

This again reminds me of some of the aliens in Star Trek or other movies where the aliens are supposedly advanced in their development with giant heads (a nod to intellectualism) and quite androgynous (a nod to social constructionists). The end goal is the removal of all gender, since gender is a prime limitation for us physically, intellectually and spiritually.

You may have heard the statement, "The future is feminine." As feminine primacy will run the show soon. However, even that sentiment is beginning to change to "The future is non-binary." This means what will be running the show in the future is without gender distinctives, no masculinity or femininity.

Essentially, these statements are about what people believe about power. It is a style or perception of power that is "power-over" and "zero-sum". This is where my ideas are very different as I perceive that mature and healthy use of power is "power for" and "abundant". Zero-sum is the battle for that elusive 51%, which is only a worthy goal in sports or business, not in life or relationships since there is only so much power to go around.

It seems that our options are these;

1) We see Masculinity as an idea constructed by society, therefore we can and must socially construct it to become more befitting of our gentler, more feminine culture. As in the future is feminine.

2) We see any gender as a lower or less valued category (regardless whether it is natural or socially constructed) therefore if humans are to advance progressively, we must create a genderless society. As in the future is non-binary.

3) We recognize Masculinity as a natural given, therefore we pursue avenues of building healthy and mature men who have a strong and positive influence in our world. I would say this means the future is human. (This is the approach of Solid Man.)

The prevalent modern perspective is that nature is something to be either transcended or dominated. It is not something to be embraced, as though it is essentially defective or too primitive, even disease ridden (toxic). This mindset seems to think to embrace our nature seems to be embracing "de-evolution", becoming less human, not more. I don't believe this is true for a second, the natural world is who we really are. We become more human by embracing nature, within us and without, not by casting it aside or castrating it.

Things seem to be kind of nutsy in our politically correct world, tree-huggers demand we attend to nature, but in other categories we throw it out. We would never tell someone transitioning from one gender to the other that their (xer) journey is not a natural and substantive part of their (xer) natural internal structure, but have no problem telling a "cis" gender man that his Masculinity is not nature, but socially constructed.

Like I said, we are in a nutsy time.

> ➔ **We exist in a very confusing time when it comes to gender.**

The two schools of thought here are "Social Constructionists" who believe that gender is determined and built into a person through culture or nurture, and "Essentialists" who believe that each person has an "essence" intrinsic within them which is how their gender exists and interacts with the natural world.

The natural world is where we really fit. It is our essence. We are made of the same stuff as dirt, horses, worms or trees. Yes, we have developed culture and cities, but we are part of nature in our being or essence. We must breathe, we must eat, we must have sex and we must shit to survive, just like any other creature of nature.

> ➔ **Do we need to transcend nature, as though nature is something to overcome? Or do we need to embrace it and guide it into the maturity as it was designed?**

The truth is this, if Masculinity is a thing of nature, it does not matter what you believe, that thing deep within you is there and will come to life when you allow it to. Nature is something you cannot avoid.

> ➔ **Mother Nature bats last.**

Man Rules

Most of what is communicated in our culture about what a "real" man is, has to do with external behaviors or movements. The idea of "man-up" is just that, in certain situations a "real" man will "man-up" and do what needs to be done to fulfill the expectations of what a man is expected to do. If he is unwilling or incapable of achieving whatever desired expectation, he is looked down upon and not considered a "real" man.

> ➔ **The Man Rules are social constructions.**

These categories or rules are socially constructed aspects of Masculinity or manhood. These external expectations are what guides men to navigate life in the present culture. Men are expected to be a utility to keep society driving forward, if you do not work you are not a man. Tim Allen jokes that men only have two options in life, work or prison.

Men are the ones in conscription, ready for literal disposal in war. I signed my card when I turned 18 and even though I have never been drafted it has been an expectation in my life. The tension and strain of this reality is part of our socially constructed experience.

Even if internally I may have been ready and even desired to fight for my country, remember that these socially constructed aspects of life are just external expectations, not the reality of our core of natural masculine soul.

These external expectations are very common and are what most men think defines them as valuable or worthy. Notice who it is that determines the value of that man. Once he achieves the desired behavior or outcome, the culture (often a specific woman) confers onto him his value. It is as though she "knights" him with worthiness when he does whatever "man-up" thing that is expected. "Man up" just means conform to expectations.

The man rules are a list of externally referenced expectations that have been developed by society to direct men to become what the prevailing ideas about what a man is or what is expected of a man. A man "earns" his manhood by assuming responsibility to produce resources and/or security for society, women or family.

⮑ **The Man Rules are externally referenced expectations.**

Whatever the culture says at that point in history about what is needed from men, it creates that expectation. It may be the need for 17-year-old men blindly going into war for the Civil War or World War II, or for long-haired beatniks in the 60's and 70's being cool and open to the times, or the post-WWII dads having 2.5 kids, working hard and getting a house with the white picket fence in the suburbs or for today's flaccid, nice guy lumbersexual with his beard, glasses, flannel and skinny jeans. These are all social expectations of men at various times in history.

⮑ **For society to run smoothly, men must be a Utility.**

At any given point in history the cultural expectations of what a man is, determines what utility the man will have to keep it all going. The utility of men has been the determining factor of what is expected, and the expectations are called the "Man-Rules". This is how the externally referenced man finds his value.

The "Man Rules" or the "Man Box" are lists of things that determine whether a man is a real man or not. Here's just a few common ideas floating around in the Man Box. Notice how externally referenced these expectations are.

Here are a few of the rules;

Do what needs done to make sure your woman (or women in general) is/are happy.

A real man has high status, everyone looks up to the real man.

Be a "White Knight", protect any woman who is in trouble, especially from her abusive boyfriend or husband, never be like "that guy".

Don't show emotion; there's only 2 emotions; Angry or Not Angry.

Men are providers, not caregivers or nurturers.

Be self-sufficient, you don't need help or directions.

Men are alphas, natural leaders. Don't be a Schmuck or orbiting Beta.

Have an authoritative posture; make all the final decisions and demand respect.

Be and act physically tough and sexually dominant.

Suck it up and Get 'r Done.

Pay for the meal, every time.

Get married, have kids and provide for them.

Be the breadwinner, it's a problem if your wife makes more than you.

Restrain your masculine tendencies, because Masculinity is toxic.

Hold rigid gender roles; heterosexuality, hypersexuality, homophobia

You must have a level of high physical attractiveness; fat, bald guys need not apply.

Your posture must be aggressive and in control.

There is also the ideas that the size of your dick, or the size of your wallet, or the size of your truck, or whether you ever sit to pee (only women do that!), or whether you use a straw (because real men would not suck like a baby), if you cry at movies, the quality of your beard, or if you are always in control; all these determine the degree to which you are a real man.

> ⤳ With the Man Rules we perform what we do rather than be who we are.

Take the idea that a real man gets married and provides for kids. Often this comes from the Christian community. It is interesting that the two most important figures in the Christian faith were very real men, but neither were married or had kids, Jesus and the Apostle Paul. If neither of those men were real men, then where would a Christian man discover what it means to be a man?

Notice that almost every one of these factors is externally referenced, it's about what a man does, not what or who he is. These externals have nothing to do with the core of a man. The man can have all the externals; big beard, big muscles, bedding multiple women, big bank account, etc., but he probably is still just a boy in a man's body.

The "boy" has not built a strong internal point of reference, he has not been initiated through the Void and he has not adequately answered the five intentional questions every man needs to answer. Essentially, he has not taken his raw masculine material and developed maturity with his masculine soul.

Every man who has developed these externals and plays by the "rules" know deeply that there is something about himself that feels like a poser or a fraud. He knows that there is still something missing. That "something" is not his Masculinity, what is missing is maturity.

Maturity is when someone has moved into a next stage of life properly. As in developing from a boy (child) into a man (adult). The proper stage is what is seen as normal growth process. A two-year old would not be expected to work for a living, as a thirty-year old would not still be in Mom's basement. Our goal with this work right now is to find what "mature" Masculinity looks like, then from natural and mentoring stages, make that happen with millions of men.

There are hundreds of other external things that have been used throughout time to determine a man's value. Most of these rules are just "stereotypes" by which people create a single or shallow narrative of the masculine.

> ⤳ "A stereotype is an unreflective, self-serving generalization made by someone who is too lazy or too stupid to think carefully." Harvey C. Mansfield

The man rules are not our model or pathway into mature masculine living. The rules seem to come from some bizarre space of stereotype and caricature which creates a very limited and convoluted narrative. It seems odd to me when men repeat these rules as though they are their own rules, when obviously the rules are not theirs.

Whether it is Odysseus or Achilles on a glorious quest or a regular guy doing what the culture expects by procreating, providing and protecting, the measure of a man still is an external judgment, the rules. What you will be reading here is not about creating another external expectation. This process is designed so you can find your internal masculine soul, not pursuing what others expect or demand. Even though a glorious quest or procreating and providing may be what is in store from that internal place, it will be without the need to prove anything.

➦ **You must find your internal masculine soul.**

To get to a place of confidence in your own Masculinity, you must look deeper and consider what is rumbling around in your core. Then take that natural part of you and nurture that into strength and maturity.

➦ **Masculinity is intrinsically expressed in biology, instinct and spirit.**

The rules have led us through what seems like becoming a man is. If we do these "things" or follow these "rules", only then are we a man and are manly. It is as though being a man requires doing rather than being. We must "do" the rules not just be who we are.

This is a concept called "Precarious Manhood" where our sense of our manhood is on the edge and we can lose it with one event or even one criticism. When someone says "man-up" they are saying that your manhood is something you must earn or do. You never hear "woman up" because a woman's womanhood in our culture is based in her natural being, a woman can just be a woman.

However, it is true that more women are beginning to question their femininity and if they are "enough". It's not just men who wrestle with being. But that is a different story.

If Masculinity is something that is based in the world of external rules that we must continually earn, then Masculinity will continuously be at the whim and expectation of whatever notion the present culture has at that time and Masculinity will indeed be precarious. Your sense of self, as a man, will be precarious or fragile.

KEN CURRY, LMFT

◔ **If Masculinity is based on "externals" it will always be precarious.**

When it is based in externals, manhood or Masculinity is something to be won or achieved and not something that is the essence of a man. For all of history there have been tribes and cultures which believed manhood was something to be grasped or achieved; a "quest" for male validation. If you hear words that sound like, "a real man does…" or "a man should do…" you are listening to voices from the outside trying to dictate an external version of manhood.

Here are a couple voices which speak this fragile idea. Norman Mailer said it this way, "Nobody was born a man; you earned manhood provided you were good enough, bold enough." Or the poet Leonard Kriegel, "In every age, not just our own, manhood was something that had to be won."

The 'Man Rules' actually are social constructs. Precarious manhood exists because of pressures to be a certain way or do certain things that are seen as acceptable or were seen as acceptable in years gone by. The idea of "do this or do that" and then you will be a man, is a socially constructed pathway to keep men doing what needs to be done.

Ideas like "Gender Role Strain" or "Gender Role Conflict" exist because men have been told what is expected of them. Rather than moving from inner integrity of who they really are, they must live up to a certain code or external expectation. What creates the strain within are those expectations to be a certain kind of man that fits the ideas of society, which often is in conflict with inner realities.

◔ **Masculinity is not precarious.**

If we have to prove our Masculinity or earn it, it was never ours to begin with. I am saying it is ours from the start. It is already in there. Masculinity is something inherent in a man, not a rule to be followed, not as a utility to keep things going, not a thing to be proven, it is a solid part of a man's being, it is anti-fragile.

◔ **Masculinity is anti-fragile.**

The concept of anti-fragile means that something is not easily broken or disintegrated. The thing can withstand just about any storm or disaster. It is not fragile. It's not going to break under pressure. Masculinity is anti-fragile, therefore it is Solid.

Masculinity is not precarious, it does not crumble under "gender role strain" nor does it falter if the culture calls it toxic. Since it is "of nature" it will prevail long after whatever whim or fad of what culture "warriors" demand. Masculinity will remain long after this cultural season of disdain.

> ☞ Masculinity will remain. It will not go silently into the night.

The challenge within this Pillar is to begin to know, experience and develop a strong sense of being; that you are a man and that your manhood already exists deep within you. It is not something you win, earn or prove. It is not something the culture says to do or not to do at their whim. Masculinity is something you already have within you that you develop into deep strength and maturity with mastery.

As your Masculinity begins to solidify within you, it becomes something you are, something that is far from precarious. It IS you, in your being, not what you do but who you are. From this true narrative, you can begin to master the art of becoming good at being a man.

There is the big question, why be masculine, why even try? If I am just going to be shamed for being part of the Patriarchy, an oppressor or tyrant just for being strong and confident, why would I even want to become empowered? This is a question we need to answer. I think the answer is simply, "Because I am a man, I will be a man, I will do what a man does." Men are strong, men are powerful, men are forces for good.

To hell with whatever accusations or pressures that may be thrown at you, become the strongest man you can be.

> ☞ Maybe there is no incentive to grow up anymore. It used to be that being a grown-up, responsible man was rewarded with respect, power and deference. Now, not so much.   - Dr. Helen Smith

The less masculine a man is, the less mature he is. In this world that calls Masculinity toxic, what we need is not less Masculinity, but more. When a man moves from external references, living as others expect rather than from his core, then what he presents to the world is unhealthy, maybe even toxic. But when a man is empowered to live from the truths within, from his internal frame of reference, he will give powerful gifts to his family and community.

The Solid Man process is a project to increase masculine power in our world, to empower men. To some this seems scary because their narrative is that masculine power has been and is the problem. Or they live in a zero-sum power game which believes that if men have power then women have no power.

This comes from a very limited view of power where there is a struggle to fight and scratch for the little bit of scraps on the table. It is time to empower all humans with abundance power. There is plenty to go around.

A Definition of Masculinity

Here is Merriam-Webster's dictionary definition;

1 a : MALE - *masculine* members of the choir

b : having qualities appropriate to or usually associated with a man - a *masculine* voice

Essentially Masculinity is just qualities usually associated with a man. That's not really helpful for our endeavor because we need something more substantive or descriptive that gets to the heart of the fullness of a man.

Masculinity is defined by physical, behavioral and spiritual aspects of being. Masculinity is different than femininity in many significant ways. It is true both are human, both are of equal value or worth, both are made in the image of God and have that divine spark. In essence, Masculinity is significantly different than femininity physically, behaviorally and spiritually. Simply stated, yet oddly controversial, men and women are different.

- Men and Women are different on many levels.

Some people believe that the idea that men and women are different means that they are or will never be equal or have the same worth and value. Each are designed with the particular gifts each brings to the table, for example, men are physically stronger, and women can grow a child in their womb. These are totally different gifts to the world, but each are equally valuable from humans who are full of dignity.

- There is neither Jew nor Gentile, neither slave nor free, nor is there male and female, for you are all one in Christ Jesus. Galatians 3:28 (NIV)

One is not better or above the other, but we are different. This simple, yet complex idea is not an easy thing to put to words, especially since there is much energy and pain that many have felt over the centuries. We are different and equal.

Human complexity is a significant consideration. Who we are and how we move as humans is a mysterious thing. As soon as you define something, something else is revealed. We are physical beings, but also spiritual. We are relational beings, but also individual. There is mystery and humans cannot be fully categorized or explained.

My work here is effectually undo-able. Masculinity has tons of mystery, many things about it that are unknown or unknowable. This is especially true as each man seeks to make it real for himself. All men carry Masculinity different than others, no one is the same. My work here is to create a map that will help define clear aspects of Masculinity. Your work is to make this real in your life, however you see fit.

This effort to define and categorize Masculinity is difficult, if even impossible because of our complexity. But at this time, we need to at least make the effort, since so many external narratives are trying to tell a story about men.

There are a million ways to define Masculinity. Here's my attempt as insufficient as it might be. Actually, this whole book is the definition, but here is a sentence and a paragraph to describe Masculinity as simply as I can.

"Masculinity is a man being a man."

Or, with more words, following the Solid Man Map of Masculinity;

"Masculinity is a deep reality present within the core of every man.

It is revealed in a drive to be a generous and powerful force for good,

founded upon a solid internal integrity and identity,

expressed through purposeful and creative movement into the world,

and lived out with passion for life and relationship."

Each part of this definition reflects what you are about to read. To have a short paragraph to define the concept of Masculinity will be deficient since there is so much to it. However, this definition is what we will work with if we are going to get the words out to describe this thing called Masculinity.

> ☞ Masculinity is like pornography, I know it when I see it. — George Bruno

If I have consistency in my thinking, that Masculinity is a natural, deep reality within every man, then it doesn't matter how I define it here, it will rise up on its own and let itself be known. My work here is just to open a conversation about what it might be and how a man will carry it with maturity.

Four Foundational Thoughts

1. Masculinity is good and designed to be a force for good in our world.

Masculinity is not toxic, instead it is and has been a force for good on the planet for millennia. Read that line again. What does it feel like to read that? What reactions do you feel? To consider that Masculinity is not only good but a force for good seems completely counter to what men have been heard for decades.

It is true that men are quite aware that they have the capacity to move in immature and foolish ways, but it is those foolish decisions and not Masculinity that is unhealthy. Masculinity is good, but some of our choices, not so much.

It seems that sometimes Masculinity is perceived as a scourge in our world. You know the line, "If women ran the world then…" But the opposite is actually true, men have created, developed and maintained amazing structures, infrastructures and inventions that provide amazing luxury, safety and well-being. Men have literally given their lives for the well-being of others in our amazing culture.

There are always a few evil exceptions to the rule; Hitler, Jeffrey Dahmer, Judas, but the vast majority of regular, ordinary men get up every morning to make the world a better place.

It is those regular men who keep the lights on, keep homes heated, gets food to the grocery stores, keep your cars running, everything we take for granted in our culture is primarily kept going by men. That's just basic infrastructure stuff men do every day.

Many boys growing up today are receiving the message that they are just defective girls. Their boyishness is frowned upon and often drugged in order to keep them attentive or within certain behavioral norms in contexts that don't come naturally. The message continues to haunt us that something is wrong with boys and men. That's just not true, Masculinity is good.

2. **The definition of Masculinity must come from the inside of a man, and from the world of men.**

The voices out there ready and willing to say what a man "ought" to be are countless. The world of women endlessly talks about what they expect a man to be and do. Many men try to hear what that expectation is, only to find it is just another moving target, wavering around in pop culture. It's just another external expectation.

➲ **Men have given "Woman" the position of Judge. She has our approval in her hands, dispensing it or withholding it at will. We are at her disposal, when will she slam the gavel?**

Over the years somehow men have allowed women to determine our value. In doing so we have subjugated ourselves to their opinions of what is good or bad in a man. The outcome has become generations of men trying to figure out the formula; what does she want? Trying to figure it out is like trying to hit a moving target in the dark. Like the proverbial blind squirrel who might get the nut, once in a blue moon we hit the target and get the pat on the head, good boy. This is not how our value, nor the definition of Masculinity is found. We've been chasing our tail too long, or other tail we're chasing?

Men have Masculinity in their being, we know it's there. We must unapologetically discern it for ourselves and then live it out like we want to, not like what is expected. The definition must be from us. Not from "oughts" or expectations.

➲ **Live out Masculinity like you want to.**

It is important for each man to determine his own pathway to becoming the man he is. Your own personal variables will guide you to mastering YOUR own personal Masculinity. There are many consistencies within the definition and make up of what Masculinity is, but it will be your journey to take these core aspects and make it your own.

⌐▶ **Be unapologetic about being a man.**

It is surprising to me how many men are ashamed or apologetic about being men, or being a masculine being. It's the idea that women are the pinnacle of creation with beauty and grace, and men are lower beings; ugly, earthy and clumsy is wrong.

It's like a comparison between elves and orcs. It is true that women carry beauty and grace, but men carry significant attributes as well. We equally bring goodness and beauty, just in completely different ways.

This volume will give my perspective from one man to another. Take what I bring, consider what resonates with you and create your unapologetic unique version of good, healthy Masculinity. It will come from within you. Let it come alive.

Defining Masculinity is the work of men and must be developed from the hearts of men. Feminism has had her say, it is time for men to speak.

3. **In order to become what it has been designed to be, Masculinity must be released, not restrained.**

Most of what is taught about Masculinity is that in order for it to be lived out in healthy ways, it must be restrained. We must keep our sexuality at bay, it is like a wolf we cannot feed, or we will at once become uncontrollable in our appetite unfettered like Mr. Hyde. We must restrain our deep selfishness because it will cause us to become unreliable as we pursue pleasures and neglect our wife and family or anything good.

There are many ways that we are taught that restraint is our primary movement toward maturity. Restrain your intensity, your anger, or your aggression. Pay attention and restrain your attention to this or that. Restrain your desires, your passions, your wants and emotion.

Don't get in "trouble", don't be in the way, get the job done, don't make waves, keep the world turning. Your desires are a pathway to sin and evil, so because sin is crouched and knocking at the door, keep it restrained and in its cage where it belongs or literally all hell will break loose!

You've gotten messages like this from all the contexts in which you have lived; Family of Origin, school, workplace, church, and from our culture. Everything screams "Restraint!", "You can't do that!", "Get in line and fly right!".

This is where men set aside their emotional process, whether that is deep feelings of grief, loss, sadness, pain or excitement, passion, or happiness, you mask or restrain your emotion, since emotion gets in the way of efficiency.

> ◔ **The rule is, don't express emotion, there's a job to do!**

A proposition I will posit here is that most of the problems men face exist because we are trying to restrain powerful and significant aspects of our soul, which only results in increased anxiety, more anger and unleashed compulsive behavior.

We must release these significant parts of who we are as men. This sounds counter-intuitive because of all the messages we've been taught, but this is the way of freedom. The more freedom a man has, the greater strength and power he has, and the less he gets caught up in the things that entangle and enslave him.

Many men are aware that they are indeed capable of powerful actions that can be dangerous and even violent. It is true, we are dangerous beings. We have the capacity to destroy, harm and even kill. Even though we hear of killings in our 24/7 news cycle media, it rarely happens, and the vast majority of people do not commit murder or violence.

In the Narnia story, Lucy asks Mrs. Beaver if Aslan is a "safe" lion, she answers, "Oh no, he is not safe, but he is good." We are capable of violence and we are dangerous, **and** we are safe. Sounds like a crazy statement, but it is true, since men are good.

I know I have these truths within me; I am sexual, I am strong, I am passionate, I am dangerous. I also know it is not the job of culture or anyone else to restrain me, except myself. I will choose my own time to express and release, I will choose when I restrain and hold myself back. I will move with wisdom and self-control.

> ◔ **I am the only one who will restrain me, I will choose.**

When a man lives from an externally referenced position of others restraining his person and his power, he experiences feeling tied down and cornered. For an unobserving man, this results in counter reactions of anger, intensity and disruption. Consider how you have felt when you were restrained, rather than free. Your goal here is to take back your own personal control choosing your own restraint.

This endeavor is not about restraining Masculinity, but about releasing Masculinity in all its fullness and glory! As you hear that Masculinity has glory, that probably gives you some reaction, "Really? Masculinity has glory? That's not what I've heard."

We haven't heard much good because the definitions/expectations of Masculinity that have been developed in the past half century are reactions to things like the "evil" patriarchy, men/boys are thrust into contexts in which Masculinity does not thrive, and the expectations of what women want in a man change constantly. It is time for men to be released into freedom.

4.   I do not have a feminine side. No man does.

The idea that a man has a feminine side, or a woman has a masculine side is an idea that has been conjured up. I do not believe it is truth. It does have some deep roots in Eastern religion (consider the Yin/Yang symbol) and in Jungian thought about animus and anima, but it is just an idea.

I think in our culture today this idea has taken on greater energy because it lays out a strong comparison between the masculine and feminine, building upon the idea that men and women are the same.

It is usually convoluted into the idea that good characteristics are feminine (nurture, verbal communication, care), and bad characteristics are masculine (aggression, intensity, sexuality). Like so many ideas that are coming out of our culture these days, this is BS.

Rethink the idea that the masculine is only aggressive, promiscuous, hard, assertive, risk seeking, frank, leader, not emotional, aloof, distant, boastful, forceful, loud, laconic, stoic, rational or abstract and that the feminine is; caring, faithful, soft, sensitive, security seeking, indirect, seeking company, warm, emotional, sympathetic, modest, persuasive, quiet, loquacious, complaining.

What if all these things are just things and they are things that a man or a woman would just do like a man or a woman would do them? Or things any human does at a particular time. A woman leads like a woman leads. When she leads, she is not being like a man, she is a woman leading. A man nurtures like a man nurtures. When he nurtures he is not being like a woman, he is nurturing like a man nurtures.

Usually when a woman is trying to do something like a man does anything (or a man trying to do something like a woman does anything) it becomes a strange caricature of reality. When a woman tries to be competitive like a man it is strange looking, like she is trying to live up to some contrived expectation, but to watch women compete like women in any sport, its beautiful and works just fine.

- ➔ **These behaviors are just things, not particularly masculine or feminine.**

I am a very nurturing man, ask my kids, and I have done it like a man would do it, with muscles; big hugs, wrestling and with a compassionate voice. It is good nurture and it's been a huge part of my masculine presence with my family.

So, when I am doing certain things that have been connected to the feminine, I am not acting from my inner feminine or feminine side, I am just doing that particular thing as a man would do it because I have no feminine side.

Let's look at these behaviors; competitive, stoic, dominance, and aggression. Both men and women can do these things and be this way. There are important times in life when you are required to call these forth in your life no matter who you are. Competing for a job? Go for it. Need to get a job done? Be stoic, suck it up and get r done. Need to set good boundaries with your family of origin? Get dominant and tell them what is right. Need to stand up for someone? Open up a can of aggressive whoop-ass. Who the hell cares if you are a man or a woman, all these previous situations are not about gender or sex, it's about what needs to be done by whoever is there to do it.

I would imagine this idea may have some reaction within you. Consider what that might be and why it feels that way. What idea have you been believing? This idea may resonate with you. Consider what life looks like if you move in ways that have been thought to be feminine in a masculine way.

It is interesting that some will say no one has any feminine or masculine side, because there is no such thing as masculine or feminine, these binary ideas are just "social" constructs. Eliminating Masculinity and Femininity is what is called a non-binary opinion or narrative describing sexuality and people. As you have read, I don't agree with this, because I think Masculinity and Femininity are nature in essence, not socially constructed. So, I do have a Masculine side.

How has this idea been formed in your head? What reactions do you have? What if it is true that you have no feminine side?

What is Masculinity? Is it a concept or idea created, developed and therefore able to be changed or modified at the whim of any fad or politically correct movement? Is it a natural state of being within a man that has inherent qualities that needs to be mastered in maturity?

> ☞ Competence is Power, Mastery is Great Power, Creation is True Power.

What you will be reading from here may give you a sense of incompetence, that you are not good at this, yet. This is a reasonable feeling, since most men have not seen or been given a good model of Masculinity. In a sense we are all beginners. So, to begin to gain competence and eventually mastery, it is important to start with humility and the "beginner's mind".

As with learning anything (a musical instrument, a martial art, an academic pursuit, etc.) you begin with incompetence and inexperience. You are a rookie. Be ok with that. You won't get far without it. Even though your Masculinity is natural and deep within you, it will still take the 10,000 hours (or more) to gain competence. Like walking, it took a while to get that down.

Now let's get into the details of the deeper and full definition of Masculinity as it is described in the world of Solid Man. In this work you will learn concepts you've never probably attached to Masculinity, so open your eyes and enjoy the journey. We'll start with a few unavoidable contexts and then draw out for you the Heart of Masculinity with the two significant paradoxes that define our journey as men. We will discuss more about this when we talk about mastery.

Here are five things I say are true about Masculinity;

Masculinity is a thing. It has substance, it has definition and it is real.

Masculinity is a mystery. It has aspects that are unknowable or undefinable.

Masculinity is nature. It has biological, spiritual and behavioral form.

Masculinity is good. It is a force for good in this world.

Masculinity is yours. You define how it will be carried out in your life.

And one thing about you;

You will master your Masculinity only by following the deep internal truths that already exist within you, not by doing or being what others say or expect.

Questions; Where do you fall on the spectrum of Nature v. Nurture, or the concept that Masculinity is a brute fact, or an idea created by culture? How so?

How have you been caught in the trap of believing Masculinity was determined by external constructs like how you look, the size of your penis, how many women you had sex with or your status (money, job, car, etc.) rather than internals like integrity, courage, passion, personal strength or wise choices and actions? Describe this.

To what degree do you believe Masculinity is essentially good or do you believe it is inherently toxic? Assess this from a personal place, you as a man, ok or not ok? Explain why you think this.

With the definition I present here, what comes to mind and what reactions do you have?

Of the four foundational facts, which seem to capture your attention and have the most value? Which ones don't seem to fit with your worldview? *Masculinity is good, Masculinity must be released not restrained, Masculinity must be defined from within, A man has no feminine side.* write your rebuttal, why you disagree and what your proof is otherwise.

When you consider the idea of mastering your Masculinity, what seems like an obstacle, what seems do-able, what seems exciting?

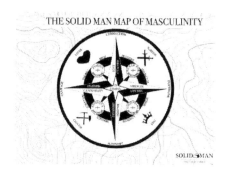

THE SOLID MAN MAP OF MASCULINITY

SOLID MAN

3 Tension and Paradox

We will begin our discussion of Masculinity with the context within we find ourselves. I will be laying out the constructs of the ongoing and ever-present existence of tension in our lives and the two paradoxes that exist which create that tension. These realities are central to understanding the essence and being of solid Masculinity.

Tension

From Merriam-Webster;

Definition of TENSION

1 a : inner striving, unrest, or imbalance often with physiological indication of emotion

b : a state of latent hostility or opposition between individuals or groups

c : a balance maintained in an artistic work between opposing forces or elements

2 a : the act or action of stretching or the condition or degree of being stretched to stiffness : TAUTNESS

b : STRESS 1b

Tension is that sensation or condition of stress or opposition. Tension is at the very core and essence of Masculinity and manhood.

Being a man (even being human) requires that we live in the fullness of the tension that exists because we live in a world that exists in tension continually.

For the exercise of uncovering the deep aspects of Masculinity we must understand that humans live in tension. The very central context in which Masculinity is designed, matured and experienced is tension. We are continually stretched, challenged and tested in this world and we must accept that condition if we are to live in the fullness of our great masculine soul.

⮚ Tension is the context of Masculinity.

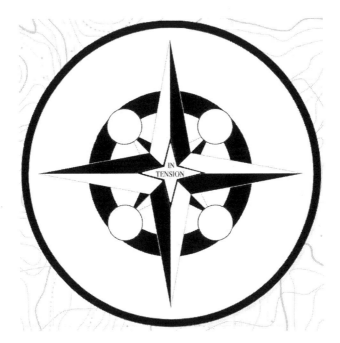

In Tension, The Inescapable Center of the Masculine Life

The Map of Masculinity begins with the idea of In Tension directly in the center. We live In Tension all of our lives and it is important to "Intentionally" stay in it. Most men are uncomfortable with tension and do everything they can to avoid or "pull the plug" on it. Staying In the Tension is how you will grow as a man.

Tension is that thing that is in the air when someone speaks the unspoken, it is the awkward silence, it is the moment before you hold someone accountable, it is when you question what is going on. Often you can feel it as sexual tension as uncertainty of where a moment is going to go increases. Its why it is hard to get up in the morning. It is when you have no idea what the outcome will be. Tension is what makes stories, movies or books good, it holds your attention. Tension creates attraction and connection, when you experience it with someone.

Tension Element #1; Nature and Culture

The first point of tension is the crossroads between our nature and our culture. I have alluded to the fact that Masculinity and being a man is nature. We are as much of nature as the elusive wapiti or a beautiful kestrel. Our DNA is in us as much as it is in any other animal or plant for that matter. We were designed to live in nature and nature is inside of us.

The tension comes from the fact that now, predominantly, we live in culture. Culture is not natural. Culture is a human design to keep out the chaotic forces of nature from harming us. To me the best illustration is The Netherlands.

The Dutch engineers have held back one of the most powerful forces of nature at bay. With their minds and ingenuity, they have kept the forces of the ocean tides from reducing their land to a salt flat which would be under water most of the day.

Consider how culture is designed to keep nature at bay. Whether it is consistent electric service, running water, warm heat in winter, cool air in summer, roof over your head, supermarket shelves full of food; we have created systems which hold back natural forces.

> ⮂ **We are Nature.**

Culture sets itself against any natural phenomenon that seems to be destructive or negative to itself. Culture sets itself against nature, that's what it does. It exists to keep Nature's dragon of chaos at bay. This is one reason why it seems like culture is pushing so hard against Masculinity. Masculinity is one of those awesome and powerful forces of nature.

Masculinity and Chaos have had a beautiful dance throughout the ages. Our legends and stories talk about men slaying the dragon, defeating evil or conquering huge obstacles. This is us doing what men do, creating environments of thriving and beauty. We have been created to defeat chaos, create systems of well-being and bring about culture.

But now, we live in a time where Masculinity has worked itself out of a job. In the "first" world, men have done too good of a job creating and maintaining a world of security and safety. We've pushed back chaos to a degree where we rarely experience it and when we do (Hurricane Katrina, Indonesian Tsunami) we are shocked that things like this can even happen, "We should've known!"

Now, it seems Masculinity is dispensable, and we don't need it. When we were reliant on low-tech agriculture or needed men to fight and die in low-tech warfare (Civil War, WWI and WWII), culture was glad to have Masculinity at its disposal, literally.

➔ Masculinity is a hammer seeking a nail in a house that has already been built. – Jack Donovan

Now that it seems that in this culture, we don't really need Masculinity, culture quite ungratefully, has begun to engineer ideas and shaming boundaries to keep men and Masculinity restrained or eliminated. Our strength and power are no longer needed, so what do we do? This is a great aspect of tension; how do we maintain a strong presence of Masculinity, while integrating into our culture in mature masculine ways?

We are now just "Utility" keeping things going and afloat. We maintain and support. There's not much building, exploring or expanding going on. It's pretty much just keeping it all together and working. Just be the utility and everything will run just fine. Do your duty and keep is all running smoothly.

The blogger Dalrock puts it this way, "Feminism is the assertion that men are evil and naturally want to harm women, followed by pleas to men to solve all of women's problems." This is the absurdity in which we live; it's a man's job to keep it all working so that everyone does just fine, while at the same time we are labeled as toxic.

In the future, there will probably be a day when the "shit" hits the fan or Armageddon happens, then everyone will be ready to embrace Masculinity. Is it our destiny just to sit for now, holding fast; in preparation for that day? Recent movies show dystopian futures usually with a tiny badass young woman dominating the scene; the 110 lb. babe smashing a 245 lb. musclehead to the ground, we all know how that would end in the real world. And in reality, we all know if things really fall apart, we will need men.

Could there be a vision for a masculine person to live with presence, strength, confidence and mastery without the apocalypse?

Is the best we can do is just sit and wait, holding fast to our masculine self with hopes of one day being useful? This is the "utility" thinking at its best.

> ➔ Solid Man creates a vision for Masculinity that transcends being a "utility", it is so much beyond what most of us can conceive.

Solid Man exists to develop millions of empowered men who have significant influence within their families and communities, where men are an ongoing force for good and beauty in the world. That masculine presence will change all aspects of the well-being of people and the planet, just because we are here, and we are empowered.

Tension Element #1; Integrating our Natural Masculinity into Man-made Culture is a tough balance at times.

Tension Element #2; Void

I have spoken about this at length in Pillar 2; *Embracing the Void*, but our lives as human beings are profoundly lived out in the presence of uncertainty, limitations, emptiness and the ever-haunting specter of death.

We live in the Void and it is inescapable. Of course, as you learned in Pillar 2, we do millions of things to avoid the Void. We learned that our initiation into manhood depends on our decisions to embrace any Void construct that exists in our lives and move through it with intention and persistence.

> ➔ The Void creates powerful men.

The Void creates tension, and it actually is tension by definition. Since I have spoken of this at length, here we will just be reminded of the powerful context of the Void in our lives as a great source of tension.

Tension Element #2; Embracing the Void is essential to living in Tension and brings growth like nothing else.

Tension Element #3; Time and Space

The third contextual element has to do with categories of immanence or the here and now. Awareness of the limitations of time and space are essential in order to learn how to explore and experience Masculinity.

Time waits for no man and it keeps on ticking, ticking, ticking into the future. There is no escape. We will age. No matter what we do, we will continue to move to the next moment. We have no control over time. All we can do is be conscious of the present, make choices in the present and experience the present. Being present in the now is required in order for Masculinity to be experienced in its fullness.

➔ **Presence is the essence of being masculine.**

Space is another major limitation. Spatial realities face us every day; gravity, matter, distance, energy, etc. We are limited by the concrete forces around us. At its core, Masculinity is very aware of the physical nature of our world.

The masculine is very physical and aware of strength, pleasure, obstacles, challenges, force and all the other categories linked with space. To fully understand Masculinity, you must understand how it interacts with the physical world.

Our tension is simply that we know we are bound in time and space, that we are vulnerable to disease, death and the loss of things that we love. Our awareness of the potential disintegration of all things real and meaningful, coupled with the desire to live, thrive or just survive is part of our ongoing tension.

It is a major pitfall to not live in the Present, when we worry about the future, fear about something that may happen, regret from the past or paying penance from actions in the past keep us from living in the present.

Tension Element #3; Accepting the limitations of time and space creates very healthy Tension and opens up possibilities for play and adventure.

Tension Element #4; Source and Abundance

The fourth element of tension has to do with categories of transcendence or those things that seem to be out there or beyond the here and now. We all start life thinking we are the center of the universe. As we mature, we realize that we are part of something much greater than ourselves. There is something going on in the universe that totally transcends us.

Remember, this world is not what it seems. The journey of discovery needs the ability to see behind or through what seems to be obvious. Allow yourself the opportunity to see what is really happening around you.

Step through the wardrobe, take the red pill, go down the rabbit hole, walk into the wilderness; do whatever it takes to allow yourself to see beyond, so you can break free from the limitations of whatever mindset is enslaving you. Here's a clue; we really are in a battle for freedom. A certain kind of Matrix does really exist which binds the hearts of men and desires to keep Masculinity from freedom. Feel the tension?

- ❧ "Welcome, my son, to the machine." Pink Floyd

We are so caught up in the story we are being told, but there is so much more that is beyond, there is so much more. What is that something or someone that is the Source of life? Each man must find his Source, the place from which true life comes. Since life is so much bigger than you, to become the man you've been designed to be, you must find your Source. Once we anchor to the Source of true life, we are ready to build solidness into our lives from a place of humility and gratitude. Since I have spoken of this in Pillar 3, I won't go into depth here, just know it is a huge part of our life tension.

A posture of humility and gratitude is necessary in order to fully experience the journey of the discovery of Masculinity. You are not the end-all, but you have been invited into a life like you never imagined. One of the greatest perversions of humanity is a life centered only on itself. The Latin term for this is *incurvatis in se*, a life folded inwardly upon itself. This pattern is seen in sociopaths, narcissism, non-empathetic postures and even in the nice-guy and ass-hole jerk.

Masculinity in its fullness is best described as *excurvatis se*, or a life turned outward, toward others and toward adventure. C.S. Lewis said that "Humility is not thinking less of yourself but thinking of yourself less." When you are able to balance inner and outer, you'll be moving ahead.

- ❧ Masculinity is fully expressed when it is internally referenced and externally expanding.

Our world is a world of abundance which provides so much wildness, beauty and goodness, engages fully with your Masculinity. You are along for the ride and your Masculinity is the activator for full enjoyment and experience.

When we live in scarcity, as opposed to abundance, our lives become small and inward.

- ❧ With Scarcity there is never enough, with Abundance, there is always enough.

Living with an abundance posture while anchored to our Source will be a core posture for us to maintain while we live in the tension of life. You will find how powerful your life can become when it is expansive and turned outward.

Often, when men hear the language of a Masculinity turned outward that we are primarily supposed to live for your woman. While women are a significant part of our lives, they are just a part of life, not life itself. If your woman becomes your purpose, your drive or your primary focus, your life will be very, very small. As we will discover the expansive life is so much greater.

Tension Element #4; Maintaining a life of Anchoring and Abundance are avenues of navigating Tension.

Just being alive creates tension. You have been born into a situation, a family of origin, a certain culture, a specific historical moment that brings the tension in that moment. You have been born with your specific limitations with your abilities, IQ, gender, finances, and looks. You are a certain race, which depending on your specific culture or moment in time is a bonus or a detriment. Life is not fair and therefore not for the faint of heart.

➔ **The Masculine thrives when things are not fair.**

Tension is any kind of obstacle or resistance you may have in your life. The Void creates these obstacles and resistance, its uncertainty, limitations, emptiness and death are guaranteed and provided in abundance. Being masculine requires you to embrace this resistance and tension. This is how a masculine being lives, is developed and strengthened, finds maturity, and eventually masters his own life. Like the Void, tension creates strong, confident men.

➔ **A Masculine soul develops, gains strength and matures In Tension.**

The fact that life is not fair is a truth that tension will be your guide through life. As a masculine individual, embracing tension and allowing it to be central to your experience is where our masculine soul develops and takes flight. Now let me introduce some very specific categories of tension that you knew were there but may not have had words for them.

The Two Paradoxes

The two Paradoxes (or Paradoxen for Brian Regan fans), are the most significant elements of Tension in the life of any man. And for our creation of a definition as we develop our Map of Masculinity, we will place tension at the very center and the two paradoxes span out from the x and y axes.

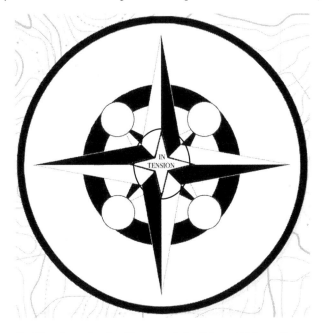

In Tension: At the Center of the Map of Masculinity

Masculinity is expressed and defined by concepts that seem counter-intuitive. This is why true Masculinity has been so elusive. Most of what we experience or what we have been told about Masculinity is only from one of two poles and therefore what we have here is a limited or only a partial view. This is true especially because what has guided us so far is external expectations instead of internal realities.

> ᕗ We have only seen true Masculinity in part.

Much in our culture seems to desire the elimination of tension, as though everything needs to be "non-binary" in order to be acceptable. This thinking is rather absurd since life and nature are binary in just about every way thinkable; dark and light, life and death, strong and weak, even conservative and liberal are in a beautiful binary dance. As in masculine and feminine, one does not exist without the other.

◔ Paradox describes the condition where two truths which seem mutually exclusive exist at the same time.

Since the binary nature of the world often exists in paradox, any true idea of masculine nature requires the exploration of the two main paradoxes of living, risk and relationship. That's where our exploration of Masculinity starts.

◔ The two main paradoxes of living are Risk and Relationship.

Since Masculinity exists in the tension of paradox, we must explore the paradoxes to fully experience Masculinity. There are two primary paradoxes which we will explore to help us understand Masculinity; Relationship Paradox and Risk Paradox.

◔ Embracing Paradox creates tension, and tension makes life fun.

These paradoxes represent the deepest tensions in which Masculinity exists. To understand Masculinity, you must understand the tension. The masculine is called into four seemingly irreconcilable points in each present moment. It is in this tension that Masculinity is developed, is defined and thrives. The men who do all they can to escape, divert or reduce the tension of life, will never experience the fullness of Masculinity.

The men who embrace tension will find their soul and then begin to master life and Masculinity. Because it is so important, I'll say that again; The men who do all they can to escape, divert or reduce tension of life, will never experience the fullness of Masculinity.

The men who embrace the tension will find their soul and then begin to master life and Masculinity.

◔ We are called into four irreconcilable points of tension in every moment.

To make this more understandable and memorable, using these paradoxes we will map out a simple structure as we define Masculinity. I will use an X-Y axis chart that shows the central concepts of Masculinity.

◔ Masculinity finds light in the dark, creates safety in danger, creates something out of nothing, and brings justice when there is none. Masculinity is a force for good that brings life to the world.

The Risk Paradox

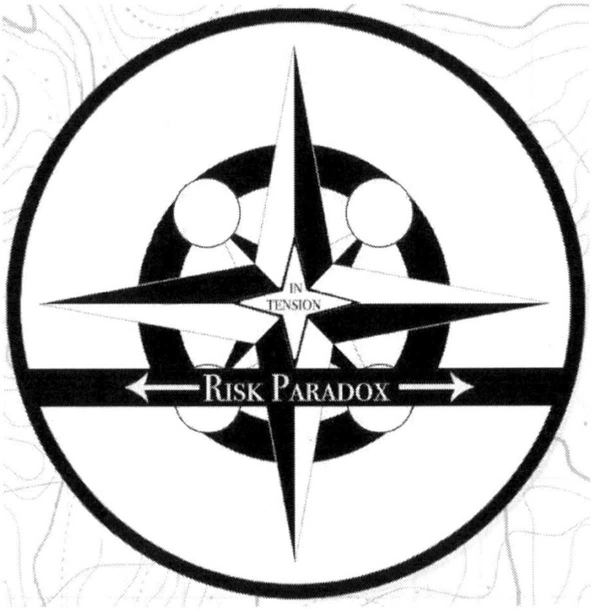

The Risk Paradox

The "Risk Paradox" represents the fact that life is about Risk. As much as we might want to hide or escape it, the truth is this; life is uncertain, the future is unknown, and you really don't have much control over your life at all.

Life is risky, full of peril and danger. Every time you step out your door you are taking a gamble. Actually, it is more dangerous to be in your house as most accidents happen in the home! What we want to do is balance the Risk versus Reward equation to make sure we are accomplishing what we want and need in a wise fashion.

- **Danger and Death are everywhere, you cannot escape Risk!**

Again, from Merriam-Webster;

Definition of RISK

1: possibility of loss or injury: PERIL

2: someone or something that creates or suggests a hazard

3 a: the chance of loss or the perils to the subject matter of an insurance contract; also: the degree of probability of such loss

b: a person or thing that is a specified hazard to an insurer

c: an insurance hazard from a specified cause or source - war *risk*

4: the chance that an investment (such as a stock or commodity) will lose value

Notice that Risk is peril, potential loss, or hazard. It means you could lose, lose something valuable, be rejected, or even die. Risk is Tension and Tension is Risk. We can do all we can to decrease Risk, but it will always be crouched at our door.

➔ **Life is Risk; security, for the most part, is an illusion.**

Since more accidents happen inside homes, even getting out of bed is a risky endeavor; stepping down the stairs, getting in and out of a bathtub, using a ladder, driving your car, things we do every day are some of the riskiest parts of life. We become numb to those facts, because if we dwelt on the danger, we would logically never even get out of bed. Where, coincidentally we would end up dying.

➔ **Manliness is confidence in the face of risk.**
   - Harvey C. Mansfield

Risk is an essential part of life and therefore a core part on the Map of Masculinity. The Risk Paradox is a powerful aspect of human life, so it is one of the two central structures lining out the map. Risk is one of the two most powerful aspects of living and so it is the "X" axis on the map.

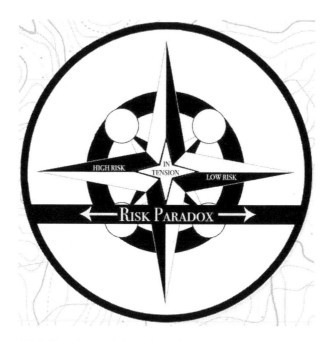

Risk Paradox; High Risk and Low Risk concurrently

On the right side of the "X" axis is "Low Risk" and on the left side is "High Risk". In the center is our good friend In Tension, the experience and context that exists as we live out life while embracing the two truths that life is both Low Risk and High Risk, simultaneously.

Even though the category of Risk is central to Masculinity and men throughout the ages have been purposefully engaging in risky behaviors, Risk is usually not specified as a primary component of a man's life. However, to really understand men, you must understand how men interact with Risk and how Risk is central to Masculinity.

Consider all the ways men engage with Risk; sports, challenges, adrenaline seeking, engaging with nature, dangerous work, pushing limits, exploring the unknown, initiating sex, entrepreneurial ideas, investing in markets, or facing rejection are all are aspects of High Risk.

On the right side of the Risk Paradox is "Low Risk" where we see men have the security of knowing that we have a certain level of strength to "hold down the fort" or "secure the perimeter". It is in a man's nature to spend a significant amount of energy creating a peaceful environment where everyone is safe and secure.

We will use strength in any form; intellectual, financial, physical, volitional, personal, cunning, intimidation, whatever, in order to provide "Low Risk" environments for ourselves and those we love. The Low Risk side is called Fortitude.

> ➔ **Men pursue Fortitude, it is what we do.**

Strength and security are good, but only half of the equation. Many men will live in the secure side because the other side has to do with Vulnerability and Vulnerability often seems like death. This is true, Vulnerability does push into the fear of possible death, it's High Risk.

Sometimes men choose to embrace Vulnerability, but usually we are thrust into it, when we can't avoid it. And it is here that we truly find out who we really are. The world of High Risk and Vulnerability is where we find out our greatest fears about ourselves and where we settle those questions as well; "Am I a coward?", "Do I have what it takes?" or "How will this end?".

Embracing Vulnerability is essential to developing and discovering your true masculine heart. Embracing Vulnerability requires Courage, wisdom and intent. There is not a man in the world who looks down on Courage. As you will see Courage is one of the Cornerstones of Masculinity.

> ➔ **Our strength is only developed and realized in our Courage.**

Even though life is uncertain, death seems to be at our door constantly, and we feel vulnerable often; the world still is amazingly abundant in the depth of our experiences. When we face our fears and push forward with courage we experience the most amazing things life has to offer.

Consider your experience when you faced Risk in a position of Vulnerability:

When we asked our future wife out for a date or to marry you,

when you took the shot to win the game,

when you went out for the team,

when you took the new job,

when you confronted your boss,

when you asked for a raise,

when you drove too fast,

when you signed up for a real poker tourney,

when you stopped a bully,

when you asked your dad about his mistakes,

when you said what you were feeling,

when you said what you needed,

when you stood up to someone,

when you confessed a wrong and asked for forgiveness,

when you said what needed to be said,

when you set a boundary,

when you told the truth,

when told your secrets,

when you said what you believe,

when you climbed the rock,

when you jumped off the rock,

when you hiked into the wilderness,

when you faced your demons,

when you said, "I am proud of you", or "I love you",

when you stood in the way of danger,

when you yelled "NO!", or just said it calmly, "no."

when you told your mother that something was not ok with you,

when you told your story to a good group of men,

when you shared your lunch with a homeless brother,

when you held your woman accountable for her foolish behavior, when you held your woman,

when you gave away your last dollar,

when you asked for help,

when you raised your hand,

when you said hello,

when you went to the doctor,

when you went to a counselor to unpack your childhood trauma,

when you let tears flow at your grandad's funeral,

when you said, "I was wrong",

when you were discouraged and kept going,

when your alarm clock rings and got up one more time, One. More. Time.

It doesn't matter what you believe about Vulnerability, any way you slice it, we are vulnerable often in life. Maintaining masculine Strength and security in life is essential and facing Vulnerability with Courage is where true masculine Strength is expressed and developed.

We love the videos of men doing insanely risky behavior; flying in a wingsuit through a small archway, insanely fast motorcycle racing on the Isle of Man or even the exciting pull of NASCAR or UFC. We are intrigued and respect the fact that some guys have the balls to do that. We look up to those who have the nerve to start new businesses and start stuff from scratch, from just an idea or vision.

Wisdom does have a part to play here. Is the behavior just stupid like Russian roulette? That is just gambling with your life. Or is it a good calculated risk that is dangerous, but still play? The fact that I might die is what actually makes it fun. I personally have known a number of men who have died rock climbing and some who died in skiing accidents here in Colorado. I respect that they were out there doing what they love, it makes for a passionate life.

If they were not doing what they were doing when they died, they would not have been living life to the full and that is what men desire.

As those things are risky, they also are vulnerable. They place a man in a very precarious and vulnerable position. Whether we experience it in exciting risky behavior or in our primary relationship, Vulnerability is a primary aspect of Masculinity.

☞ The Risk Paradox means we are Strong and Vulnerable at the same time.

The development of the Risk Paradox in our lives combines two aspects that seem like oil and water, but fit hand in glove. The tension that is created between High Risk and Low Risk experiences in life is one powerful place where Masculinity is discovered, defined and lived out.

The Risk Paradox recognizes the fact that healthy humans are at once Strong (holding Low Risk with incredible Fortitude) and Vulnerable (bearing High Risk with openness and Courage). We are at the same time Strong and Vulnerable, this is the Risk Paradox.

☞ Risk provides the masculine with a true playground of real living.

The Relationship Paradox

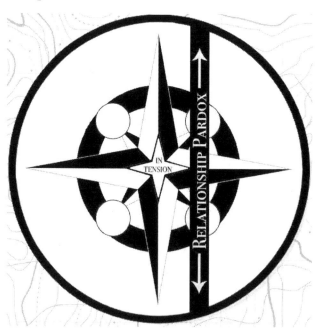

The Relationship Paradox

This paradox requires that we understand and recognize that we have been born into relationships, our relationships often define us, relationships are why we have been made and relationships are what move us forward toward true mature Masculinity. We cannot escape the fact that we are designed for relationship, it defines a central aspect of our humanity.

Today it seems science recognizes that most of the natural world exists in relationship. We exist in a world where molecules, particles, animals, chemicals, people and systems interact with each other at all times. Whether it is atoms, energy, body parts, riparian ecosystems or meteorites plummeting into the gravitational field of the Earth, everything is in relation to something else and somehow to everything else.

> ☞ Relationships are everywhere, just like we cannot escape Risk, we cannot escape Relationship.

As humans, we are inherently relational. Whether you believe it is because it is the way our species has naturally survived over millennia or this is the way we are because we have been made in the image of a relational God is irrelevant, relationship is a real and central aspect of being human.

It is one of the most significant categories in our lives. Again, I am having fun building the love between creationists and evolutionists!

Relationships provide a context for survival. Relationships meet deep internal needs. Relationships create cooperative human systems to increase well-being. Relationships force us to grow up and mature.

Where Relationship becomes a powerful aspect of tension is that it exposes us to the two most powerful human drives; Autonomy and Connection. Those two drives create the other significant Paradox; The Relationship Paradox.

The Relationship Paradox recognizes the fact that healthy humans are at once connected (part of a relational co-op; family, community, country) and autonomous (an individual, differentiated being). We are at the same time attached and detached, this is the Relationship Paradox.

> ☞ The Relationship Paradox means we are attached and detached at the same time, we are at once connected and autonomous.

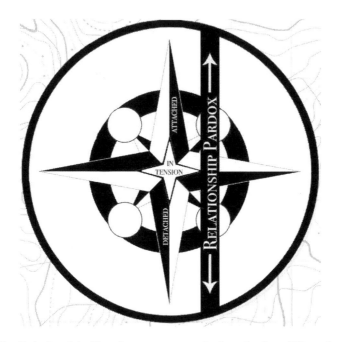

The Relationship Paradox; concurrently Attached and Detached

On our map, the Relationship Paradox is the "Y" axis. On the top line of the Relationship Paradox is Attachment, our connection with other people. On the bottom is Detachment, which is Autonomy or our ability to differentiate from others. Even reading the words Attachment and Detachment probably creates tension and questions.

Like I said, these are the two most powerful drives in the human life; the drive to be connected and the drive to be a differentiated self are inescapable. That defines this paradox, these two truths existing at the same time. How can we live with both simultaneously? This is the relational tension Masculinity is developed and revealed.

This Paradox also describes the two most significant fears of every human; Abandonment or Absorption.

 ᢒ **Our two greatest fears are Abandonment and Absorption.**

Abandonment is the fear of being rejected, left alone or not belonging. It is the fear that I will be alone in the universe. This fear is the one fear that drives just about every unconscious human decision or action. As you move toward maturity, knowing this truth will guide you well, you'll see clearly. This fear exists because we have a deep desire and need for Connection, it is essential for human surviving and thriving.

➔ **The fear of abandonment exists because we need attachment.**

Absorption is the fear that my "self" or my being will be lost, and I will no longer have any power to be me and move with any freedom. It is the feeling of being sucked into something that will take away your sense of "you". This is why someone would be hesitant to commit to marriage, or why it is so difficult for some to pull out of their Family of Origin systems because they've been sucked in so deeply. This fear exists because we have a deep desire and need for Autonomy.

There are many men who as boys were forced into a relationship with their mother as what is called a "surrogate spouse". The father was deemed as a distant, possibly abusive man who did not meet the perceived needs of Mother, so she opted to use the son as the one to meet those needs and to have someone to hold her pain and protests. The son becomes the "golden child" or "Mama's Little Man" or any variation thereof. The point is that he loses (or never had) his own self, it has been fused into the mother.

A similar dynamic happens if both parents are absent. The child becomes a "parentified" child, becoming the adult figure and caring for the younger or more anxious siblings.

This too, is losing themselves and being absorbed into a system that needs them to be a certain role. To get healthy in these types of scenarios it is essential that you do the work to detach and begin to build your own true self and identity.

➔ **The fear of absorption exists because we need detachment.**

A significant part of developing a solid core of Masculinity is to balance the two urges of Connection/Attachment and Autonomy/Detachment. The majority of relational problems occur with an imbalance of these two concepts. We usually get into situations where we have too much of one and not enough of the other.

We may be "co-dependent", fused or overly connected to others in a very needy way. Or we may cut-off, withdrawn or stonewall relationships, keeping people at arm's length or even across the country. A balance between these drives is central to healthy human relationships and is essential for healthy Masculinity.

Our drive for Autonomy is the need to be fully and freely who you are with your own, true authentic self. It is to be differentiated from others as you discover who you are, what you want and need in life and begin to identify and pursue your passion and purpose in your life.

Our drive for Connection is the desire to belong. Connection with others is one of the most profoundly pleasurable experiences life has to offer. Belonging, companionship, touch, interaction, support, have all been proven over and over to be an essential need of human existence.

Healthy relationships require the balance in the Tension of Autonomy and Connection. Your relationships are the perfect context for practicing being who you really are. As you start developing integrity and being truly yourself, you will place yourself in a position to attach to others without losing your sense of self.

➜ **Attach to others without losing your self.**

The balance of these concepts varies between different cultures as well. Some cultures are very strong on the side of community or family, there is a kind of social identity where the individual to differing degrees, is absorbed into the group.

Other cultures lean toward the side of individuality where your own identity and pursuits are more geared around personal desires, not necessarily for the good of the group.

Regardless of your cultural background or family of origin, you will experience the tension with living in balance between these concepts.

➜ **Build a balance between Autonomy AND Connection.**

It may feel daunting to start being who you are and saying what you need; you are changing the system and people may not like it at first. They may push back. But you must hold your integrity. This is one of those counter-intuitive paradoxes; developing your solid identity is the ONLY way to experience true relationship and intimacy.

With different cultural variables, how does your heritage play into this for you?

It seems that the perception of Masculinity is that men are not very relational, more on the autonomy side of things. It is the stereotype of the strong, silent type or the love 'em and leave 'em playboy type. These are just caricatures of imbalanced masculine.

The truth is that men are equally as relational as women, we just do relationship like a man would do relationship. Our goal for true Masculinity is to develop a healthy balance between Connection and Autonomy. This is what the "Relationship Paradox" is about.

⮑ Without Relationship or Risk the masculine isn't much.

The masculine soul is actuated, is developed and thrives within these two beautiful paradoxes. We live in a world of Risk and uncertainty; therefore, we must navigate life with a balance of power and courage. We are relational beings and the balance of Autonomy and Connection is essential to the development and expression of the masculine.

Questions

What do you think of when you hear the idea of In Tension?

In what ways are you uncomfortable with tension?

How do you usually pull the plug when things get tense?

When you consider the Risk Paradox, where you are strong (Low Risk) and vulnerable (High Risk) at the same time, how does that fit with what you've been taught?

As you think about the Relationship Paradox, in what ways have you been stuck or caught up in one side or the other?

What do you think of when the challenge is as much leaning toward detachment as attachment?

Which of the fears, Abandonment or Absorption, has had more significant impact in your life?.

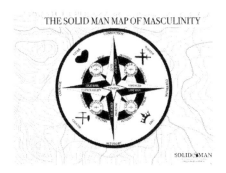

4 The Four Cornerstones and The Four Currencies

The Four Cornerstones of Masculinity

The Four Cornerstones are concepts that create the foundation at the heart of the masculine soul. As the "cornerstone" in a building is the primary part of the foundation of that building structure, these "cornerstones" are primary parts of the structure of Masculinity.

Each of the Four Cornerstones are directly related to one side of the two Masculine Paradoxes.

On the Low-Risk side of the Risk Paradox we find the cornerstone of **Fortitude**.

On the High-Risk side of the Risk Paradox we find the cornerstone of **Courage**.

On the Detachment side of the Relationship Paradox exists the cornerstone of **Autonomy**.

On the Attachment side of the Relationship Paradox is the cornerstone of **Connection**.

> ➔ The Four Cornerstones upon which Masculinity is built are; Fortitude, Courage, Autonomy and Connection

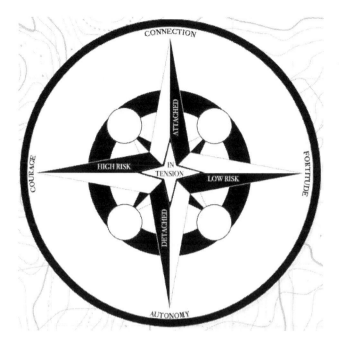

The Four Cornerstones of Masculinity

It is essential for any man who desires to develop his masculine heart to engage in these four concepts with intent and purpose. The work must be done to explore the essence of each cornerstone, deepen understanding of these concepts, evaluate the degree to which these exist within you and embrace personal practices which move you toward a full mature masculine presence in the world.

↷ Remember this: "Masculinity is a deep reality present within the core of every man. It is revealed in a drive to be a generous and powerful force for good, founded upon a solid internal integrity and identity, expressed through purposeful and creative movement into the world, and lived out with passion for life and relationship."

Cornerstone #1 – Fortitude

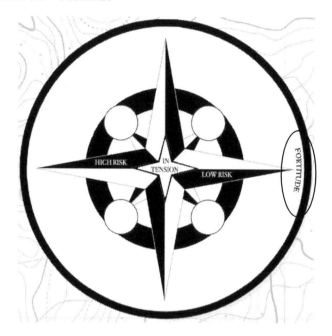

The Cornerstone of Fortitude, on the Low-Risk side

Found on the secure or Low-Risk side of the Risk Paradox, is Fortitude. Fortitude is a word which means what it says, a man is a "Fort" or a "Fortress". There are places around the world that are named for being (either in history or presently) places of protection and military might, places like Fort Collins or Fort Sumpter.

I remember walking on the grounds of Fort San Felipe del Morro in Puerto Rico. Here was a place set in the stone at the entrance of San Juan Bay designed to keep any ship that came near under complete control. In a very strategic position and with more than 400 cannons and other armaments it had been a place of strength and might protecting Puerto Rico for centuries.

A fort is a stronghold, designed to protect, hold fast against attack and be an impenetrable force against other forces that come near. It is closed off and built up "against". It is strong. It is imperturbable. It is unshakeable. This is Fortitude.

> ➷ Fortitude is closed off, walled up and strong as hell.

Fortitude is an environment of Low-Risk as it holds space that is safe and secure. Fortitude uses wisdom to make choices that are conservative and safe. It is powerful and protective. Fortitude is not open, nor is it vulnerable and only vulnerable if it might bring more strength through collaboration, but even then only so far.

⮞ **Fortitude is Strength.**

Strength is core to a man's life. Men have been designed for Strength. Strength is a man's glory. Strength is the ability to be free from external influence, to influence/change the world around you and to protect those you love and care for.

Fortitude is played out in two arenas, the physical and the psychological/spiritual. You will want to be as strong as possible with your body in the physical arena, and you will become powerful with your internal core. The Solid Man Process is geared toward making you into a beast with internal strength, where not many things will shake your core.

⮞ **Fortitude is powerful.**

The physical is External Fortitude and the psychological/spiritual is Internal Fortitude. Both are required to be a man of Fortitude.

The masculine is by nature very linked to the physical world. While our muscles and body are significant expressions of Strength, our voice is potentially even more powerful. As a man ages, his Strength transitions from his muscles to his voice; where wisdom and mastery of life gives him what some call gravitas, true influence.

⮞ **A man's Voice is powerful.**

A man with substance can rein in a troubled moment with a strong "No." His voice can be commanding and influential.

His voice can bring wisdom and restraint. We can teach, influence and bring life with our voice. Voice is a part of our Strength that has been forgotten or disregarded often.

Your Voice will only be strong and influential if your core is strong. A strong core is internal Fortitude; a core identity, worth, values, character and confidence are deep, immovable and unwavering. A man who has this, has a strong influential Voice.

⮞ **From the beginning to the end of a man's life, strength is central.**

Since Fortitude is a posture of being closed, this is often an aspect of the masculine that is seen as bad or even toxic. That is just wrong, every person on the planet has enjoyed the shelter of a strong masculine presence during their lives, or they have longed for it. The closed off Fortitude of the masculine soul provides some amazing benefits to all who rest in this safe harbor.

As Fortitude is closed to danger or threat, it is open to a select few to be within the confines of the safety of that fort. We will talk more about who is able to rest within that Strength. Not everyone has that privilege.

☞ **Not everyone has the privilege of resting in your Fortitude.**

Cornerstone #2 – Courage

On the High-Risk side of the Risk Paradox is Courage, the next Cornerstone.

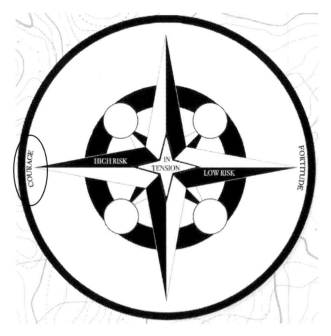

The Cornerstone of Courage, on the High-Risk side of the Risk Paradox

Courage only exists in the face of Vulnerability or danger, so Courage is found in the world of High Risk. Courage is the ability and willingness to confront fear, pain, danger, uncertainty, or intimidation with intentional action or voice.

Physical Courage is holding fast in the face of physical pain, hardship, death, or threat of death, while moral Courage is the capability to act rightly in the face of opposition, shame, scandal, or discouragement.

Courage is universally seen as a deeply respected masculine trait, often because it is expressed with selflessness and purpose. While a man often may be willing to face physical danger (either to protect or for adventure), many men do everything they can to avoid emotional or personal Vulnerability, which is a lack of Courage. Like I said earlier, men enjoy and respect watching men do highly risky behaviors, even if it just for the fun of it. Most of us have done things we look back on as something thrilling that we actually survived, with a sense of accomplishment.

Men respect courage and whatever form it takes we respect it and often look at it with admiration. We feel a sense of pride and self-respect when we face our deepest fears. Remember that Courage is not the absence of fear but standing strong in the face of fear.

Men will maintain what seems to be what could be called stoic strength, but sometimes it's a submission to fear of exposure or being found to not be good enough. It is just withdrawal from a situation where I might be found out. Keeping myself from being exposed or seen for what I really am is not courage, it is allowing fear to rule me. It takes Courage to allow yourself to be vulnerable, to be seen or possibly fail.

➔ **Courage is Vulnerability and Vulnerability is Courage.**

This is where many men reject the concept of Vulnerability as a part of Masculinity. There is a reason to reject Vulnerability, but only if there is no balance with Fortitude. A man with Vulnerability and no Fortitude is not being masculine, just as a man with Fortitude and no Vulnerability is not as well. The disdain for Vulnerability exists when it is seen as weakness and many men in our culture have chosen to be submissive and weak, this is weakness, not Vulnerability.

➔ **Vulnerability is not weakness.**

Some reject the idea of Vulnerability if a man seeks to be vulnerable to achieve a woman's endearment or validation.

I would agree here. If that is the reason for engaging in openness or vulnerable expression of emotion, to get a woman to like you or be attracted to you, that is the weak and pathetic posture of an orbiter.

Anything done with the hope of acceptance or approval is weak. That is not the Vulnerability I am speaking of, that is just submitting yourself to her judgement.

For men, Vulnerability is not weak, it is a courageous choice to be open and exposed to potential harm (either from relationship or adventure). Living a mature and healthy life with vitality requires periodic and timely choices of risk, openness and exposure. We will talk shortly about how and when a wise man spends his valuable vulnerabilities. Just so you know, it is not often and with very few.

◌ Vulnerability is not Strength.

Some see Vulnerability as Strength. This is an absurd thought. The definition of Vulnerable is that you're in a position of High Risk. When you're Vulnerable, you're exposed to potential harm or damage, either physically or emotionally. It is inherently placing yourself in a position of exposure. This is not a strong position. However, the ability to choose to live openly, wholeheartedly and exposed to possible hurt is Vulnerable, it does take Courage, and Courage reveals a type of internal Strength.

Some men have no interest in building their lives on the Fortitude side of the equation, as though Strength and Power are a toxic parts of a man. These men seem to be willing to complete the castration process themselves, hopefully only figuratively, but none-the-less they eliminate a significant aspect of the masculine soul. This is a distortion of Masculinity as much as the man who is hyper-masculine with only Fortitude without taking the risks of Vulnerability.

Wisely choosing to put yourself in vulnerable situations is risky, but life-giving. It is interesting that forgoing Fortitude is also a move to get women to approve of you, that just doesn't work. You will eventually be rejected and even ridiculed by those you thought would approve of you. The doormat gets no respect.

◌ Being vulnerable does not mean being a doormat.

There are many contexts in which a man will experience Vulnerability; pursuing intimacy with your spouse, playing with your kids, grieving at your grandmother's funeral, pride with your child's accomplishment, revealing your dark secrets to your closest friend, giving a toast at a wedding, feeling deeply when you learn you have cancer, starting your new business, or experiencing the incompetent feeling of beginning to learn a musical instrument or martial art.

Vulnerability is all these things and all the categories I mentioned a few pages ago when I was talking about exposure and Risk.

Since we are alive, we will be vulnerable. You will have health problems. You will age. You will have relationship issues. Life will fall apart at times. If you do all you can to avoid any vulnerable situation or any Vulnerability, you will remain closed off to the richness and fulness of life.

☞ **Courage is impossible without Vulnerability.**

Courage is living with a life of openness, engagement and availability. It opens you to abundance and vitality. As Fortitude is Closed, Courage is Open. The balance between the two IS the tension of the Risk Paradox.

☞ **Courage is required to experience the fullness of Masculinity and life.**

As stated earlier, life is unfair. We've been born with limitations, some more than others. When we choose ownership, responsibility and agency rather than victimhood, then we can begin to move with Courage in the most vulnerable parts of life and experience our masculine self.

Vulnerability is seen as weakness in our culture. Placing yourself in a position of risk where you are at the mercy of others is insanity to most men. Vulnerability is openness, transparency and exposure. It is leaving yourself open to attack, indefensible. At first glance, the last thing any man in our world would intentionally allow himself to be is Vulnerable.

Contrary to the cultural viewpoint, Vulnerability is one of our greatest allies in the quest for integrity, solidness and healthy relationships. Vulnerability is actually a display of what's really under the hood, true strength and manhood.

Vulnerability is the true show of internal strength. A man who is unable to be vulnerable is actually showing weakness and fear. He believes he will die or be hurt if someone rejects his true self, he just can't handle difficult situations or potential pain.

A strong man can open himself with Courage and confidence, knowing he can withstand anything, even rejection or an attempt at shaming.

Cornerstone #3 – Connection

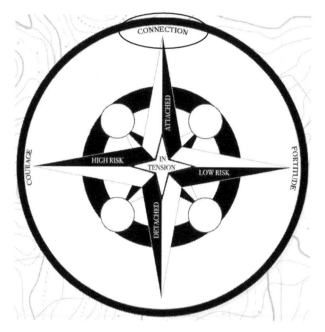

Cornerstone of Connection, on the Attached side of the Relationship Paradox

Connection is interaction with others where you are respected, loved and wanted. Connection exists when other people know your story, accept you and are in this journey with you.

Connection creates what I refer to as "entities" that don't exist if there was no relationship; a family, a marriage, a community or village, a tribe, a church, a team, a band of brothers or a group of friends. These are entities that have personality and substance.

A couple who are married has two people (entities) who come together as "one" to create a new entity, the couple. Then they may add others, whether that's kids or friends to develop their community (a bigger entity). The defining factors of a relational entity is people and connection.

➣ Relationship connection is one of our primary needs as humans.

Since it is so important, we will be fearful of rejection or abandonment if people see who we really are. When we don't believe we are ok, acceptable or worthy (when shame defines you) we will do relational backflips and contortions to somehow keep connected without letting ourselves be known.

We will sell out ourselves in order to be accepted or belong in relationships. We may wear masks or develop a false persona in order to fit in. We may trade our integrity for connection. We will do what others want. We live to please. We will give up ourselves to keep the peace or try to get what we need.

We do not reveal our true selves because we believe we will not be accepted if people knew who we really are. We live like a chameleon until Toto pulls back the curtain and we are exposed for who we really are, which at first is terrifying, but is actually a very good thing.

We know this is a sham to begin with; I am not presenting my true self, so even if they do accept me, they are not accepting the true me. That connection is based on a non-reality. Relationship will not truly exist until you present your true self.

⤳ **Connection is impossible without Autonomy, being my true self.**

This is another place where Courage is part of our masculine endeavor; allowing your true authentic self to be seen and known.

As you are able to be you, you can then build the relationships you need, so you can thrive.

Connection is developing and experiencing meaningful relationships, support, community, belonging, camaraderie, intimacy, being known, accepted, and liked. Whether it is expressed in your sexuality, family, gang, or political party; Connection is absolutely important for the human soul.

The tension between Autonomy (being my true self) and Connection (letting my true self be attached) is necessary for the masculine soul to become strong and mature.

Remember how science is beginning to notice how everything is in some kind of relationship? Everything is connected. We cannot escape connectedness, we will be connected. Our task is to take those connections and choose how you will develop them; healthy or unhealthy, loving or abrasive, distant or close, it is our choice.

Many men seem to be choosing to keep from relationship or commitment. It makes sense when you know that a prime driver in a man's decision making is the concept of Return On Investment (ROI). The ROI is an important consideration when choosing to marry or make a family. In our culture today with a high rate of divorce and the very negative outcomes, men seem to be thinking twice if it will achieve for them the return they want, since the odds are not very good.

This is where the Commodities come in; with whom, how, and when will I spend my precious and limited Commodities? This is a huge question of ROI. What or who will get me the outcome that I want from my investment? Or is that even possible?

Cornerstone #4 – Autonomy

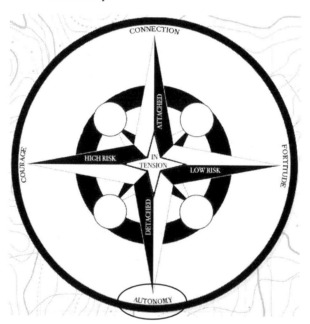

Cornerstone of Autonomy, on the Detached side of the Relationship Paradox

The Cornerstone on the Detached side of the Relational Paradox is Autonomy. This idea of being Detached seems odd to many people since we all know that "No man is an island." While that is true, we do indeed need others in our lives, this is the tension that is created by having a well-balanced life. We need balance.

Autonomy is having integrity with your being. It is having an internal frame of reference. It is having the freedom to be yourself, to pursue that which pleases you and helps you thrive.

Autonomy is personal freedom, healthy true identity, authenticity, control over your own life, being an individual, and having personal power and influence.

Autonomy is resistance to tyranny, fighting for what you know is right, doing what you want, having your own desires and opinions, being your own person. Autonomy is being a complete, whole person who does not need external validation or control.

Autonomy is differentiation. The concept of differentiation is central here. Differentiation is a high-falutin' word that just means being able to be who you are, know and say what you want and have a plan for where you are going. Do you remember Pillar 3? It's the five questions you answered. Differentiation is just being able to be you, being able to answer the questions, "Who am I?" and "What do I want?" within a relationship.

Differentiation is opposite of being absorbed or enmeshed into a relational system which operates where the members of that system need to "lose" themselves into the system to keep the system running. For Trekky fans, think the Borg where resistance to being absorbed is futile. For those who have seen their share of chick-flicks, think "you complete me". It would be any situation where you lose your "self".

⮞ **When you lose your "self" you lose it all!**

Enmeshment is the same as co-dependency and it is not healthy. If you lose yourself, your sense of identity, your needs and wants, your dreams and purpose for another person or to keep the group happy, you're screwed. You've lost the battle and the war.

As I have already alluded, many of us were raised in enmeshed family systems that required us to be a certain way to be acceptable or to belong. If we made waves or had a differing opinion, we were shut down or even rejected. We had to fly under the radar, be a good kid, don't make waves, keep mom calm, get good grades, win at sports or just blend in to fit in.

For those of you who have broken free from these systems, Autonomy has been hard-earned. Most of us have stories of how difficult it has been to break free or how it still haunts us.

Consider your present primary relationship. You've been reading this material because you want life to be different. You want change. But since your relationship was built on your former way of living, i.e. not differentiated, your changes now may not be welcomed. This is part of welcoming tension into your life. You are shaking things up by creating more Autonomy or differentiation in your life.

The hope is that your partner will come along with you, which usually happens especially when you are building differentiation in them. But sometimes things fall apart. That's a bummer since you really care for them, but facing that possibility is inevitable if you are to be the person you want to be. As you grow, this could happen with your spouse, friends or your family of origin.

> ☞ Autonomy is being who you are, telling your story, and living with authenticity.

As a Cornerstone, Autonomy requires that you gain some very personal internal strength, that's was a big part of Pillar One. If you need a refresher, go back and read Pillar One *Awakening the Internal*. You have been designed to move and live fully from an internal point of reference. Once you have been able to detach from needing others for your sense of self and worth, you will be able to attach in healthy ways.

> ☞ To become the man you want to be, you must first be Autonomous.

The Four Currencies of Masculinity

A "currency" is medium of exchange. You have one thing and you can trade it for another thing that you deem as valuable (or more) as the thing you have exchanged. We do this every day. We will take a dollar bill (deemed as valuable as that day's rate would have it) and exchange it for whatever we might need at that moment.

Commodities are similar to currencies. Currencies are a represented item (a dollar has no actual value, except for what it represents). A commodity is the raw material used in exchange for currencies that you can then trade for whatever you see as valuable. I'll use those two terms interchangeably.

If you've ever played a game like Pit or Settlers of Katan, you know what it means to trade commodities to get what you need to win. It's the same in the commodities market where things like corn, ore, wood, or wheat are traded for money, other commodities or something valuable.

Transactions happen in business and relationships all day long. Here it is important to understand and notice what a man has as Commodities (raw materials) that could be traded or exchanged for what he wants or needs to thrive. Understanding the nature of these transactions is necessary so you can achieve your goals and live well.

Initially it is important just to know that as a man you have significant Commodities. The Commodities are those things you are able to give to others or exchange in order to increase your well-being, to experience the fullness of life or to provide for those you love.

The Four Commodities which are in our Masculinity on this map with which we can give, or trade are; Strength, Vulnerability, Freedom and Love.

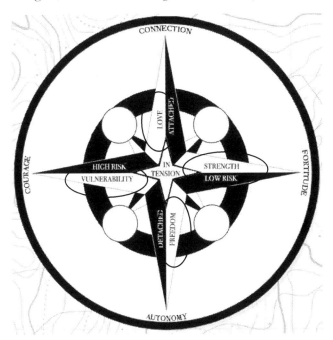

Four Commodities of Masculinity; Love, Strength, Freedom and Vulnerability

On the Fortitude side of the Risk Paradox is where we find the Commodity of Strength. On the Courage side of the Risk Paradox we find the Commodity of Vulnerability. On the Autonomy side of the Relationship Paradox exists the Commodity of Freedom. On the Connection side of the Relationship Paradox is the Commodity of Love.

◌ **The Commodities are the currency of the masculine life.**

Your personal boundaries will allow you to budget your commodities and use them with wisdom and choice. A man with no boundaries (boundaries reflect your values and moral compass) will spend his currency willy-nilly and be left with nothing in the end.

> He is a fool who allows others to determine how he spends his resources.

See your Commodities as personal resources. You only have so much bandwidth. You only have so much to spend. Where, when, with whom and why you spend them must be given significant consideration.

Consider that you can only care for only a certain amount of people or causes. Not only is it OK to only care for those closest to you, it is essential. We do not have the bandwidth to care for every problem or for every person. You must be able to accept the fact that you really don't care enough for some things, for some people.

> If we really cared about everyone, we would never even register feelings or microaggressions or First World problems because our brains would be blown out from watching Third World ultraviolence. We'd be watching and liking and sharing nonstop videos of prison rapes and basement executions and reading stories about sex slavery and child prostitution. We'd be OUTRAGED at the injustice of it all, 24 hours a day, 7 days a week.   - Jack Donovan

Often you will be drawn into care for some cause or person. This is when you must consider deeply if this is one of the few things you will give your time and energy to. You know the dog commercials which rip your heart out, or the guy at the intersection who looks way down on his luck, or the way that the media will portray some people as victims to try get you to change something about your way of life.

It is ok to say, "I don't care." It's ok to prioritize your values. I do care for those that are very close to me and I will spend my currencies on making sure they are doing well. I will choose a few causes that I will support and some people I will help, but when it comes down to it, for the majority of humanity, I just don't care enough to do something. I CAN'T care for everything. That sounds cold, but it is the only way to roll, since we have limited resources.

Since we only have so much bandwidth, we must use our currencies with great discernment and Wisdom.

Remember, you will choose who and what you want to choose to use your valuable currencies on and when you want to use them.

The Value of the Commodities

One of the greatest stories of commodity is the story of Jacob and Esau. They were twins and Esau had been born first, with Jacob close behind. This meant, as the first-born Esau would receive the whole inheritance from his father Isaac. As was the way it was in those days, he would essentially get everything.

Jacob, who was devious, caught Esau in a moment when he was hungry, very hungry. After Esau had returned from a long hunt, Jacob offered Esau a bowl of red lentil soup. Taking advantage of Esau's hunger, Jacob got Esau to agree to release the inheritance to Jacob by exchanging the soup for the inheritance. Esau's hunger was satiated, but Jacob (through some other events as well) received the inheritance.

So many of us are like Esau, we will sell off something of exceeding value for something fleeting like food, sex or validation. Most of have done this. When have you sold your soul for something fleeting? I'm sure you have a story about that.

The goal here is that you will not only think twice, but with great consideration only choose to spend your valuable commodity with wisdom. Will you sell your soul for a "bowl of chili", a short-term gain in a long-term game? But she was so hot! or they said it was a once in a lifetime opportunity, or it was the next big thing!

As I outline the four basic commodities, consider how valuable they really are. They are as valuable as an inheritance. Spending your commodities wisely will get you what you want in life. Spending them foolishly has the potential to destroy you.

> ➔ **How you spend your commodities will determine outcomes in your life.**

Another question is, "Who will I spend my currency on?". Our choices of who we allow into our lives is important as we move forward as a mature man. There are many people who would just as well use you and abuse you. Some people are like that, but some people are solid gold. You must choose wisely.

KEN CURRY, LMFT

Find people with great character, reliability and grace, then make them part of your tribe. Find people that you trust, that you are glad they are on your team and have your back. Innumerable are the men who have chosen the wrong woman because they did not vet out her character and her ability to be held accountable.

These men seem to be strewn all over the landscape, broken and deflated. I have assisted many of these men in reclamation of their lives. Getting their life back is possible, but they have paid a difficult price.

⮥ **Your Commodities are way more valuable than you realize.**

Strength

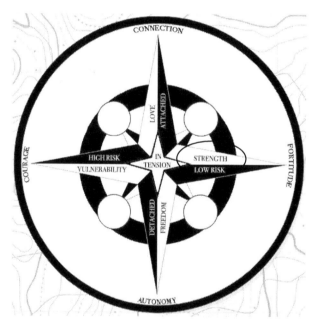

The Commodity of Strength

Strength is the Commodity at the Low-Risk side of the Risk Paradox. Strength is the right-hand of Fortitude. As Fortitude is the experience and producer of power and safety, Strength is the go-to. Strength is power. Strength is the ability to get things done. Strength is influence and capability.

As with any Commodity, we only have so much Strength. We are limited in our musculature, in our skills, in our capacities. Our voice only has so much influence or reach.

Consider your muscles. The physical Strength of any person is limited. The strongest man in the world can lift a three-hundred bound dumbbell with one arm only three times. Only three times! Even he is limited! Most men think their strength is found in their muscles. While muscles are a big part of strength, there's much more.

An unfit, flabby man can be beaten by a man with fit muscles. A man with big muscles can be defeated by a man with much skill in martial arts. A man with skill in martial arts can be defeated by a man with a good team. A man with a good team can be overcome by a man who has inspired a nation with his voice. We must build every aspect of strength. Become stronger with your muscles and endurance. Become strong in your skills. Become strong in your leadership and influence. Build your capabilities and abilities. Become strong in your voice and wisdom. All these areas are areas of strength. Build your power bandwidth. Build your Strength Commodity.

⮑ **Build yourself to have as much Strength as possible.**

The Strength Commodity is the one you can build most significantly. The others (Vulnerability, Freedom and Love) are more finite, with less growth potential. But Strength can be built, expanded and grown.

The more you build your Strength, the more you have to offer. The more you have, the more you have to spend. Or not, you can just hold on to it, so you can spend it if you ever need to. You don't have to spend it, especially not on what you don't want to.

Realize your Strength as a growing capital. As you build your capacity for earning and providing, also build your "social" capital, deepen your relationships and your networks. As a young man, you are just starting to build this as your Strength. As you gain experience and wisdom, your capital will expand intentionally.

We spend it when we go to work, because we are taking our capabilities and time, then transferring it into money so we can live. If we have chosen to have a family, we spend our Strength on providing. How we spend a commodity depends on what we value. We also spend our Currency of Strength with whomever we choose to protect.

Many men enjoy taking the role or responsibility of being a "White Knight", coming to the rescue of the "virgin" damsel in distress. "I'm here to save the day, m'lady!" Being the white knight is using your Strength to protect a woman in order to gain points (maybe get laid, maybe) or to signal your virtue that you are just that type of man who would risk life and limb for some random woman. Regardless of why a man would do this, just know, it's a choice of how to spend your Strength Commodity.

Do you really want to risk for a woman who is foolish enough to get herself in this kind of dangerous situation, a woman of questionable character who will never give you a second glance when this is done? What's the wise choice? Personally, I think white knighting is foolish, save your Strength for those you really love, for those who really deserve your protection, somebody with good character.

We could spend it on people, we could spend it on experience, or both. It is just a choice. There are many messages in our culture today that says that to be a man you must provide for a woman and sacrifice yourself for her. That is just cultural pressure. Here, I am saying a man builds his Strength and chooses when, where and with whom he uses that commodity with wisdom as he pleases, not as culture dictates. You have the choice when a with whom or even if you will make sacrifices.

⮞ **Choose where you use your Strength as you see fit.**

Your wisdom will help you decide when to spend your Strength. If you choose to spend your Strength with a woman who does not have good character or a good moral compass, you will lose the game of life. Sometimes you'll lose just about everything important to you, maybe even your soul.

If you choose to hold on to your Strength and find a woman with character or a cause with great value to you, spending your Strength generously you will achieve many things that life has to offer. But it must be done with wisdom. Then life is abundant.

⮞ Remember this: "Masculinity is a deep reality present within the core of every man. It is revealed in a drive to be a generous and powerful force for good, founded upon a solid internal integrity and identity, expressed through purposeful and creative movement into the world, and lived out with passion for life and relationship."

Vulnerability

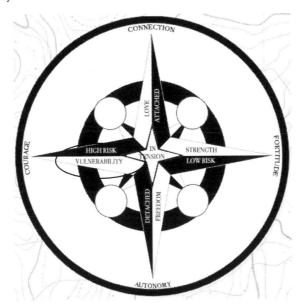

The Commodity of Vulnerability

Vulnerability is the Commodity at the High-Risk side of the Risk Paradox. Vulnerability is the right-hand of Courage. As Courage is the experience and producer of openness and facing uncertainty, Vulnerability is the go-to of Courage. Vulnerability is allowing for openness to pain, hurt and potential defeat or failure.

As is Risk, Vulnerability is placing yourself in a position of possible bankruptcy or loss. As bad as those definitions sound, Vulnerability is the pathway to so many positive outcomes in life; intimacy, depth of being, success in business, fun times or triumph in endeavors.

> ➔ **To move forward in anything, you must face Risk.**

Every historical event is filled with people who have placed themselves in vulnerable situations. We know the names of the heroes (Columbus, Shackleton, Armstrong), but most were just unnamed individuals who just went on with life, or they died right there in the trench. We know the names of Bill Gates, Warren Buffett, Edison and Zuckerberg, but have never heard names of people whose businesses failed. We know of great champions in all the sports; Gretzky, Brady, Pele, Ruth. But are unfamiliar with those who blew out their knee giving it their all in High School. They gave it their best.

We are aware that our parents had enough Vulnerability to make us when they had sex at least once, but did they have enough to hold it all together? Relationship Vulnerability is one of the most difficult arenas of Courage for men. Keeping a relationship going into deeper connection and life requires more Vulnerability than some are willing to give.

☞ Danger is Vulnerability

One way to put it is that Vulnerability is putting yourself in a dangerous position. Consider any of the potentially dangerous situations in which a man might choose to engage; rock climbing, approaching a woman for her number, taking out a business loan, getting married, interviewing for a higher paying job. Of course, you may not be killed with all of these, but the danger of rejection or loss exists.

☞ Vulnerability is the willingness to make mistakes.

We are surrounded by those who have given it a go, with all they have. And we are surrounded by those who are scared shitless to even try. Vulnerability is real, and it usually takes balls to engage with it, no matter the context. This is why Vulnerability and Courage are so intertwined.

So how do I spend this Commodity? You only have so much. You can only open yourself up to a very limited group of people. You can only go after so many opportunities. How do you choose?

Spending the Commodity of Vulnerability means that you would purposefully place yourself in a position where some of your greatest fears may be realized.

☞ What you want is just on the other side of your comfort zone. - Robert Allen

We experience Vulnerability the deepest with fear. Two of our deepest fears as humans are the fear of abandonment, rejection or not belonging and the fear of being devoured, absorbed or loss of self. As you consider where and when to spend your Vulnerability, be conscious of what you have been afraid of your entire life.

Which one has it been? Is it abandonment, not fitting in, being outcast or rejected? Or has it been an underlying feeling of being absorbed by darkness, where your sense of self is slowly being lost? Look back into your family of origin to find the clues you need to understand your deepest fears. When you understand your fears, you will understand how to move with Courage.

Courage is required to move into Vulnerability. Wisdom is required to choose how, where and when to place yourself in a vulnerable position. Do I go parachuting, free rock-climbing, ask that woman her name, share something important with a friend? Is it time to explore my father or mother wound? Any of these are choices of Vulnerability. Each choice places you in a position where you could potentially be rejected, exposed or even die.

Sometimes men have a difficult time talking about or expressing emotions. I believe most men actually do share their emotions, it is just how men do emotion is not accepted in today's society. Since men don't do emotion like women men are often mis-labeled with a concept called Alexithymia. Because we don't express emotion like women, we are seen as flawed, like something is wrong if you are somewhat stoic or pensive.

Alexithymia is the inability to identify, express or describe one's feelings. Since we have been told our whole lives to hold back or stuff our emotions, many men do struggle with doing emotion efficiently. To be integrated, a man must be attentive to all his internal processes, including emotion. We must build awareness of our emotions, build our vocabulary of what is going on inside of us and be able to communicate those emotions, so we can care for ourselves well. Sharing our emotional process is an exercise in Vulnerability.

Expressing our emotion and what we are feeling deeply exposes our inner self to potential scrutiny and criticism. Most of us have experienced ridicule and have been exposed as incompetent in this arena of life. Of course, that is vulnerable. This is why it is important to have strong boundaries around when and with whom we share these deep feelings, that is, who we spend the commodity with. Men don't share their stuff with just anyone, so when you see a man being stoic, in any situation, know that he is not spending this commodity with you, which is fine.

Danger exists in this world. Living in this world requires courage. Courage requires Vulnerability. Getting out of bed is dangerous, driving is dangerous, expressing our sexuality is dangerous, allowing anyone to see our true heart is dangerous, asking for help is dangerous; life is full of danger and vulnerability is placing yourself in any of those situations. How will you spend this valuable commodity?

First you must realize that you must have the Courage to allow Vulnerability into your life. Vulnerability opens you up to so many things in life; tell your story, be who you are, be authentic, feel, experience, let yourself be seen, develop intimacy, play, laugh, ask for help, etc.

☞ **Don't be closed off all the time in your life, just some of the time.**

Second, you must be wise with whom and where you allow your Vulnerability to be expressed. Choose well who you spend your time with, who you give your heart to and what business to start. You only have the bandwidth to give only a few people your deep self. And usually only one person gets the deepest parts of you.

☞ **Only let the closest people to you see the deepest parts of you.**

The action of choosing to open yourself to the potential of harm often seems like a pathway to death, but it actually opens you up to greater things in life. Vulnerability sometimes feels like certain death. Vulnerability feels like death because we think if we are exposed and people see the true "me" then I will possibly be rejected. Your external mask or self-protective walls will be seen for what they are.

Even though this feels tragic, having our method of hiding exposed for what it is, is actually a gift that will open our lives to true living. Once we are able to begin to live from an authentic place, as we allow the truth of who we are to be seen (which is Vulnerability), the opposite of our fears happens. We discover that good people around us actually want to be closer to us and they actually enjoy being around us.

☞ **Vulnerability is the pathway to intimacy.**

In your closest relationships, allowing yourself to be vulnerable results in relational closeness. Many of us have been closed off our entire lives because of shame and the belief that if I talk about inner struggles and experiences that I will be seen as less than or not enough. This belief has kept us from experiencing the depth that relationships have to offer.

☞ **Vulnerability is THE antidote to Shame.**

Shame is the idea that something is wrong with me or that I am inherently not acceptable. It is the idea that guilt is I made a mistake, but Shame is I AM a mistake. The more we show up in our lives and allow ourselves to be seen, the more we defeat the power that Shame has held over us. We begin to actually see that we will not be rejected, but we will be accepted and loved more than we ever knew possible.

☞ **Defeating Shame will take courage, and to defeat Shame, you must open yourself up to others, that is, be vulnerable.**

Freedom

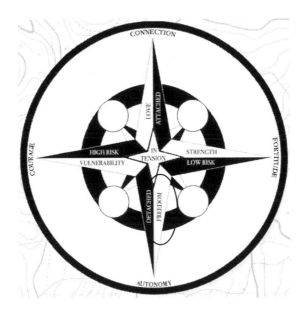

The Commodity of Freedom

Freedom is the Commodity at the Autonomy side of the Relationship Paradox. Freedom is the right-hand of Autonomy. As Autonomy is the experience and producer of differentiation and building integrity, Freedom is the empowerment of our Autonomy.

Freedom has to do with will, choice, accountability and unconstrained agency. It is having the power to pursue and do what you desire. Freedom is associated with Autonomy since Autonomy is a posture of independence, self-governance and freedom from external control.

None of us will ever have complete freedom. We live in society that has laws and ways of doing things. Some societies allow for more Freedom than others. We live out the measure of independence our society allows. Society might have some limitations, but many of us allow ourselves to be enslaved by fear or lies that have their root in our beliefs about life and who we are.

> ☞ It is for freedom that Christ has set us free. Stand firm, then, and do not let yourselves be burdened again by a yoke of slavery. Galatians 5:1

Masculinity thrives in a context with independence and the ability of self-determination. Depending on your philosophical stance, true Freedom may or may not exist in varying degrees. However, the masculine will usually push through toward whatever Freedom is available, even (or especially) if there is threat of pain or death.

> ☞ The masculine always pushes toward freedom.

There is something inside of a man which has an inherent resistance to tyranny. We strive to achieve in work, we move toward personal goals and we push to gain something better for ourselves and those we love.

> ☞ Freedom is like Power, the ability to do what you want.

Sports is a great example of the desire for Freedom. The strategy and physicality of any sport is to create a moment where the athlete achieves freedom to break free from the opponent and score. Men love sports because we love Freedom, and victory. The struggle to accomplish and win represents more than just a game, it represents the struggle in life. That's one reason sports is such a draw for men.

Understanding our deep desire for Freedom allows a deep understanding of how the masculine moves in relationship with women and the world. Look at Freedom as a Commodity, we only have so much time, energy and capability. Our day is limited by 24 hours. Our energy is limited by how much we can do before we need to rest. We are only capable of so much. Unlike Strength, which we can build, we can't really increase or expand how much time we have in a day. It's limited.

> ☞ Our Freedom is limited.

We can make our time more efficient or increase our ability to achieve more in less time. We can eliminate addictions or distractions that keep us from living clean and well which will bring more abundance and sustainability to the time and energy we have. But we are still only working with so much, and all men have a similar amount.

How we choose to spend our time, energy and capabilities is important. Who do I spend time with? What will I do for work? What do I want to accomplish in my day? Why would I want to invest so much time with that certain woman or job? What is holding me back and stealing my precious time?

> ☞ Time is a very precious commodity.

Reclaiming your Masculinity is reclaiming your Freedom. It is becoming a man who is able to do what he sees as necessary and right. It is choosing according to your internal values and moral compass. It is making the decision to thrive. Your Freedom will bring more power into your life and give you more space with which to master your Masculinity.

Love

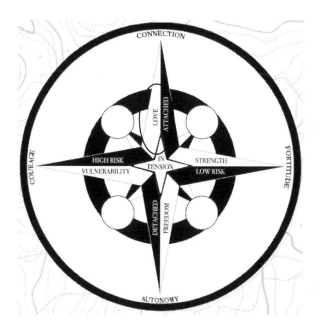

The Commodity of Love

Love is the Commodity at the Connection side of the Relationship Paradox. Love is the right-hand man of Connection. As Connection is the experience and producer of openness and building relationship, Love is the empowerment of Connection.

We have all been flooded with ideas about what Love is. It's a feeling. It's a decision. It's the affectionate feeling you have for your mom. Love is the experience when you have your favorite meal. It is the twitterpation when you fall in Love.

Love is the attraction you have with another human, when you see them. It is the nostalgia when you consider good times in the past. It's the attachment you have for your kids or friends, that transcends reason sometimes.

Love is often described as an action, where you move and give affection, compassion and appreciation. It is when you are loyal to the well-being of another. It is when you express kindness to another being, or a desire for their happiness and thriving.

Love has been described as a virtue, if not THE highest virtue. As a virtue it is goodness, honor, righteousness, dignity, kindness, decency, respectability, and purity. It is benevolence and care for others. It is generosity of the deepest kind, where you share your soul in connection with another.

Love has been described in categories of unconditional or conditional. I can give it as a choice with complete disregard to any action or way of being, totally unearned. Or it can be transactional, where the other has done something to earn it.

It could be that deep understanding you have with others, kind of a settled loyalty between family members, friends or in a band of brothers. Love is also that deep feeling in your groin, when you are horny. It is that passion that moves you to want to have sex, the urge to merge. No wonder Love has been the subject of so many songs and movies, it is in so many parts of life.

    ⟳ **Love makes life worthwhile.**

All these categories represent the Love that men experience. As far as the exercise in defining Masculinity is concerned, Love is the deep desire for connection (emotional and sexual) and the unselfish, loyal concern for the good of another.

As a Commodity, we need to understand what Love is, our capacity for Love and the ways we spend it. This is where men get really wrapped around the axle. Men through the ages have moved in chivalrous ways to get the hand of the maiden. Which is not a bad endeavor, unless she is your "all in all" or "my world" or "my density", then it is really foolish. If all your Commodity of Love is spent to get her hand, you'll regret it.

    ⟳ **Putting a woman on the pedestal is as foolish as a man can get.**

When the woman becomes your purpose, your world shrinks and becomes very small. So, when it comes to Love, don't get caught up with it being centered around just a woman. I am not saying that a relationship with a woman is not important or even primary, which it is on both accounts, but it must only be a part of your experience of life and Love.

⊙ **When the WOMAN is your purpose your world diminishes.**

This sounds like I am advocating polyamory or affairs. Not at all. What I am saying is that our expression of Love must expand greatly into our world with your purpose and passion in many other forms. Absolutely save all your sexual energy (*"eros"* Love) for your chosen woman but expand your passion and excitement for life and living to make as much of a positive impact on your world as possible. She will love you for it, most women don't like being on the pedestal, that creates too much pressure. She might think its cool for a short time, but then she will resent you for it.

Presently it seems that the expected role for many men is to rescue the single mom and take her children as your own. You must be the "good" man because her ex is a dick. This is where your value is determined by your ability to rescue and to sacrifice yourself. You can do this if you wish, just remember the Commodities you are spending are yours to choose where, when and with whom you will spend them.

You could choose to marry a single mom, that's a potentially reasonable choice. It's not a problem if it comes from a noble place of internal choice, not out of neediness or what is expected of you. It could be a beautiful thing for you to bring children under your wing who do not have a father. We chose for 8 years to do foster care and we cared for kids whose parents couldn't do it. We chose to feel real pain and loss when we gave them back after giving them deep connections. That was our chosen sacrifice.

⊙ **If you want to pay full price for used merchandise, that's your choice, just be as wise as possible.**

How do you spend your Love? This is answered by where you spend your focus, attention and resources. It is what you place as your highest priorities. Your attention is yours, no one else's. Your choice of priority is yours. As with the other Commodities, you only have so much. Where, with whom, when and why will you spend it?

There are voices which will scream at you to make them a priority and try to capture your attention and focus. Stay strong, my son. Choose ahead of time what and where you'll have as your focus, where you'll spend your passion, where you'll spend your resources.

Many times, your choice will be making a sacrifice. When you spend your currency on someone else or for a cause, you will be sacrificing something very valuable to you. It is a gift that you have to offer. Only give that gift when you want to and to ones who will receive it as it is, a valuable gift.

↪ **Your focus is a gift of your Love.**

You can choose to be a statistic like so many other men who lose their wisdom and choose to give all of this Commodity to women, with the hopes of gaining validation. Or you can be wise, hold fast to your integrity and moral compass, then choose well how to move in life with this precious Commodity of Love, with the right woman, for the right reasons.

Understanding the four Cornerstones and the four Commodities will help guide you to living out your Masculinity with intent, purpose and wisdom and guide you into deeper understanding of Masculinity. They will help you know the foundations of who you are and how you've been designed to live.

From here we will continue to build our map as we look at the quadrants which will outline the four Benchmarks, eight Muscles and four archetypes of our masculine soul. As the quadrants are explained it will become very clear to you how Masculinity has been designed to engage with our world with Strength, Vulnerability, Freedom and Love.

<u>Questions</u>

Fortitude; I am a strong fortress, invulnerable, closed and powerful. **Courage**; I face fears, I engage with life, I take risks, I initiate. **Autonomy**; I am myself, I stand on my own feet, I am complete. **Connection**; I have my tribe, I build relationships, I pursue intimacy.

Which of the Cornerstones do you want to develop further?

Strength; abilities, skills, capital, power, presence and voice. **Vulnerability**; willingness to live openly, with emotions or adventure. **Freedom**; independence, self-governance and power to choose. **Love**; passion, benevolence and care for others.

Which of the Commodities do you naturally do better at? Which seem to be difficult?

Which of the Commodities would you want to develop?

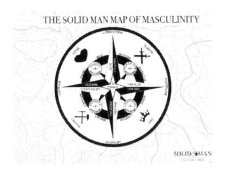

5 Quadrant One – Power For

From here I will be outlining the "Quadrants". Between each set of Paradoxes and Cornerstones is a quadrant. This is where we will further develop our understanding of the masculine heart. This is where you will discover some very concrete descriptions of the masculine soul. The full expression of Masculinity will be outlined as we unpack all four quadrants.

In each quadrant is a Benchmark of Masculinity. I learned about Benchmarks from my Dad as he taught me about the outdoors. Occasionally as we wandered through the woods, we would find a round metal marker about 4-5 inches across set in a rock or a concrete post. The marker had valuable information indicating elevation, latitude and longitude.

It was often placed at the corner of a section and you could find your bearings on a topographical map. They were there mostly for surveyors but were important for anyone finding their way.

> Remember this: "Masculinity is a deep reality present within the core of every man. It is revealed in a drive to be a generous and powerful force for good, founded upon a solid internal integrity and identity, expressed through purposeful and creative movement into the world, and lived out with passion for life and relationship."

A benchmark looks something like this with numbers stamped into it.

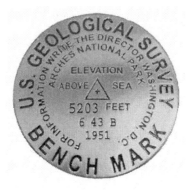

A Typical Benchmark

This was how you could know where you were in the backcountry before everyone had GPS. Presently, the term "benchmark" is used often by businesses and entrepreneurs to measure if they are up to standards or achieving what they have set up as their expectations.

It's the same concept; a benchmark is a standard or point of reference by which things are measured or judged, it is a guiding principle which helps evaluate your position, your condition or accomplishment.

"Benchmark" is a marker which shows you where you are. That may be in the backcountry or doing business on Wall Street. Here I am using this concept to give you a strong reference point for establishing and assessing where you are as you develop your strong and confident masculine self.

There are four masculine Benchmarks, each developed and born from the two of the four Cornerstones. Within each Benchmark are what I call the "Muscles" of Masculinity. The Muscles are about action and more specific "doing" behaviors, how your Masculinity moves and is experienced.

There are two Muscles associated with each Benchmark and they are like our real muscles as you will be exercising and developing them to grow them bigger, stronger and more powerful. We will have a total of eight Muscles to build as we map out becoming a strong man.

Benchmark #1 - Power-For

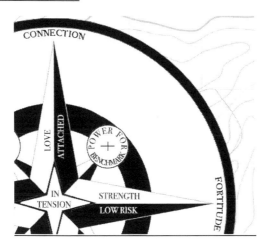

The Power-For Benchmark

At the corner between Connection and Fortitude is the Benchmark called "Power-For". Power-For is found where the Commodities of Love and Strength meet. Connection and Love on one side and Fortitude and Strength on the other. They seem like oil and water, but they come together in a very significant way.

The Fortitude/Strength side of the equation is where the concept of Power comes from. A man has been designed to be powerful and strong. He has been made to be influential, to initiate, to get things done, to work, to protect, to make positive changes in the world.

Power is the ability to be free to do something. It is the capability to do things, whether that is by influencing like a coach or a boss, or by having the personal skills to get whatever it is, done.

To most the idea of Power is an obvious characteristic of Masculinity. Increasing Strength has been a significant part of the lives of most men, whether physical, intellectual or in capability. Our increasing Strength in turn increases our Freedom, which increases our options, which gives us a good life. This is good.

Where Power goes awry is when we need to have "Power-Over" others. Tyrannical power is Power-Over. One person or system controls another person, reducing the other person's personal power and freedom. That person then has less power and must comply with the one who has Power-Over.

This type of Power is often equated to the concept of Zero-Sum. Zero-Sum is usually used with competition. There is a winner (+1) and a loser (-1), plus 1 minus 1 equals 0. The sum is zero. Many in today's culture have an understanding of Power only as a Zero-Sum category. (If the husband has Power, the wife has no Power.). It is the world of the victim and the oppressor. The victim has no Power, the oppressor has all the Power.

When the Power of one person (or system) is a controlling dictatorship, it is the Power-Over and Zero-Sum type of relationship. In history we have seen this with people like Hitler, Communist Dictators, various warlords, business monopolies and in authoritarian households (it could be either Fathers or Mothers).

The idea that masculine Power is only Power-Over has been a narrative derived from a Zero-Sum perspective to advance "equality" for women. While it is absolutely true that there have been many contexts in history where men have exerted Power-Over, both men and women can use power like this. We are all capable of using Power in unhealthy ways.

The false narrative that men are oppressors at their core, therefore Masculinity must be restrained or eliminated is wrong. While there are oppressors of any gender, most people just want themselves and their loved ones to do well. This is very true for the vast majority of men.

Even though men are quite capable of Power-Over, it is not the way Masculinity has been designed. Our hearts reveal something much deeper. The deeper and much stronger way of expressing our Power is a concept called Power-For. The power of the masculine has been designed to be FOR the wellbeing and love of self and others.

While Power-Over is for the benefit of only the one carrying the Power, Power-For is using strength and influence "FOR" the benefit of others. My Power is "for" those who may not have much Power.

This idea requires a completely different way to see Power. Rather than seeing Power as limited and win-lose (which it is in sports and tyranny), know that Power can be experienced and lived out with abundance as win-win for everybody. Everybody is empowered.

The Abundance View of Power believes that there is plenty of Power to go around. If the husband has Power, the wife will share that Power and become more powerful. As she becomes more powerful, he becomes more powerful, they become a Power-Couple. Abundance Power begets more Abundance Power, everyone thrives, there is Power for all.

⌐ Unlike Zero-Sum Power, Abundance Power is win-win.

Mature masculine Power is Abundance Power. We have been designed to become the most powerful beings we can possibly become, so that those around us can thrive as well. We are made for Power-For. Our Power is "For" others not "Over" others.

Dominance and Submission

The idea of dominance has been a part of most conversations about Masculinity. Many writers call this idea "hegemonic" Masculinity, which means it is authoritarian. The assumption is that this is what Masculinity is, that it is about dominance.

This is a faulty viewpoint. As I said before this is immature or the "Power-Over" and Zero-Sum categories of power, whether from a man or woman. Presently, in our zero-sum world, hegemonic Femininity is as common as hegemonic Masculinity.

Recently the concept of Alpha and Beta is tossed around as normal aspects of manhood; a dominant man is Alpha, and a submissive man is Beta. Or it is assumed that if one is submissive and therefore Beta, he is not really a man.

This must be part of our conversation around Power. Those who talk about Alpha and Beta as such usually think in Zero-Sum power structures. However, the idea of Alpha-Beta is a natural thing in the world of many animals and there it is not used as Power-Over.

While the alpha wolf will be dominant while the lesser beta wolf submits and shows its throat to the alpha, it is played out quite differently than how humans would do Power. The beta wolf is now in a great position to be a huge part of a great team. He may not be the top dog, but he is a huge part of the pack's success. Seems rather like an abundance view of Power.

If the alpha killed or injured the lesser wolves, there would be no pack and no survival. It is enough to know the dominance hierarchy and then move successfully in it, where everyone thrives. Sure, the alpha gets the best cut of meat and first choice in mating, but the beta does just fine. With a little patience, his time will come and all in the pack does better.

⌐ Not everyone has been designed to be the alpha, but we all have been called to be free.

If alpha means Power-Over, then the idea that all men need to be alpha is quite foolish. But if Power-For is the norm, it works quite well. Here, alpha does not have to have Power-Over (dominating) but is good with Power-For (dominion). There is no need for chest pounding or driving a lifted pick-up truck with loud pipes. True Power and dominion actually come from not needing to be dominant.

> ➔ Most alpha-ness you see is just posturing to look strong and in control.

Rather than the word "dominate", defining Masculinity, the more accurate word is "dominion". Dominion is having Power, no doubt, but it is Power to have control over your own life and Power For the betterment of those who are under your care or those you have chosen to use your commodities on.

Dominion is a place of leadership and ownership of the well-being of people within the sphere of influence of that person. It is very similar to control or dominance (that is Power-Over), but Dominion is Power -For. This man will say, "I have great power, even Dominion and this power is for the betterment of myself, my family and my world."

> ➔ A man with a confident core will probably be an alpha, but the point is that he doesn't need to be.

It is the difference between control and influence. Control says, "meet my demands!", while Influence nudges those around him toward good, calling forth health, life and beauty. Dominating is control, Dominion is influence.

A man who has a solid internal core and has built a strong self, physically, mentally and spiritually, will have an internal strength that has no need to gain status or puffed up alpha-ness. He can be OK with submitting to a coach, a boss, or God because he has an internal confidence that his manhood is not dependent on whether or not he is alpha.

> ➔ The world would be a different place if Power-For was the norm.

The humility that comes from inner strength is real masculine Power. This is another aspect where Vulnerability comes from inner Power where there is no need to be inflated by external validators. The truly masculine man is internally strong, and he respects other men who have strength. He builds up and empowers a man with limited strength to become a man he wants on his team. This is Abundance Power, this is Power-For.

Benchmark #1 Motto:

"I will become the strongest, most powerful man I can be,
so I can love others well."

Increasing Your Power

There are a number of sources of Power within each person. What we usually think of first is our Physical Power, but then there is Cognitive Power, Presence and Influence which comes out of Confidence, Competence with our Skills and Abilities leading to Mastery, and the last one, but potentially the most powerful is our Voice.

Physical Power is found in our muscles and what our muscles can do. This is a basic sense of being able to get stuff done, to achieve athletic endeavors and to possibly dominate over others. This is the Power that young men get caught up in. They think this is the source of true Power. It is Power, but a very limited source, our muscles can only do so much.

Increasing physical Power is developed in good and healthy things like exercise, nutrition, sleep, self-care and medical care. So, go to the gym, eat well, go to your Doc, take care of your body, build this great resource of Power.

Your Cognitive Power is also limited. Each of us have a certain IQ or ability to learn. But we can do all we can to make sure we get the most out of the good mind we have. Even if your IQ is not Mensa level, you can still gain as much knowledge as you can. Even if you can't read at a 10th grade level, you can listen to podcasts or audible books. Even if your fifth-grade teacher said, "you'll never amount to anything!" you can prove her wrong by believing in yourself by building your smarts.

The Power structures of Presence and Influence come from a man's Confidence. Confidence simply is knowing you're ok and that you can handle just about any situation that comes up. Having a Confident posture then gives you Presence, or that sense of gravitas, when you are in the room people sense substance. YOU are here, now.

When you have Presence, you will then build Influence, which is just the ability to nudge those around you toward greater good and empowerment.

Competence means that you are good at something. You have skill and ability to accomplish what you want. Competence creates great Power. Increasing your competence toward mastery places you in a position of even greater Power potential.

➲ Competence = Mastery = Increased Influence

Voice is probably one of the most powerful aspects of being a man. If you are able to find your Voice, master your Voice and use your Voice well, you will experience more positive power and influence than ever realized you could. Simply speaking who you truly are, what you want or need and speaking clearly from your passion and purpose will change your world.

It may possibly change the world itself. Consider how the Voice has been used throughout history to influence, to inspire, to hold to account, to call out wrongs and injustice. Consider the voices of Abraham Lincoln, Martin Luther King Jr., Ghandi or Jesus, how they have changed the course of history. Think about how the simple statement from Rosa Parks, "I don't think I should have to stand up.", changed the course of the Civil Rights Movement. Her Voice was powerful and so is yours.

The Voice has been huge in history, and it is powerful in any relationship as well. Being overt about what you want and need, speaking a clear boundary for how you would like to be treated, expressing your love or pride in someone, or even the simplest sentence, "No." are all ways of using your voice with Power. Finding your Voice and mastering it is primary with gaining masculine Power.

Limitations are at play here. We all have limitations in many areas. We have great strengths, but we have limits as well. Our work, as we build our Power, is to consider our limitations and press them to the limit, while building on our strengths. This endeavor creates full personal strength like nothing else.

While much of your focus as a man will be toward self-care and increasing your capabilities and power, the outcome of building strength is not just for yourself. Every man has a deep internal desire to make sure everyone in his care is doing well. Which brings us to the two Power-For Muscles.

➲ Power-For is significant because the Masculine has been designed to protect and provide.

The Muscles of Benchmark #1 Power For: Provide and Protect

Reflecting the concept of Power-For, the two Power-For Muscles are Provide and Protect. These Muscles are found between Connection and Fortitude and are expressed through the Commodities of Love and Strength.

The Provider Muscle

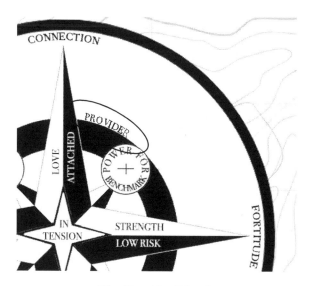

The Provider Muscle

Leaning toward Connection and Love, but still fully connected to Fortitude is the Provider. The Provider does just that; he provides. Remember that the idea of Connection could be any entity of relationship; family, friends, community or even a gang. It doesn't matter what the entity is, providing is what the masculine is and does.

A provider produces, comes up with and distributes what is needed for any given need within the group that he has chosen to belong to. The first action of the provider is the choice with whom to spend his good, hard-earned commodities.

When we buy into culture's idea of what a man is, our perspective of work often becomes our identity, we are what we do. This externally referenced perspective is what most men see as their value in the world. A man is not a human being, who is, he is a "Human Doing" who does.

Roy Baumeister says it this way, "Across cultures and throughout time, people have one expectation of all men everywhere; that is that we produce more than we consume." The Prime Directive the world has for men is to be efficient and effective. A man has to get things done in the world to make sure everyone else is ok. Which is what I earlier called being the Utility, that is, keeping the machine going, usually in spite of his own well-being.

A wise man will take the time he needs to determine if any woman, mission or group is worth his hard work and self-sacrifice. If a woman is does not have good character, is unwilling to be held to account for her poor behavior or unwilling to respect a man for who he is, she would not be a wise choice to place your commitment to Provide.

Many externally referenced men have this unhealthy desire to rescue. They will unwittingly choose women with a few kids to care for and provide since they have been abandoned. Some single moms are very good women, but the fact that they are in that situation is a huge red flag. Re-assess your "need to rescue" quotient and consider at least three more times. Be wise with who you choose.

➔ Your commodities are very valuable, don't spend them willy-nilly!

I have spoken at length in previous work how men lose themselves seeking external validation from an unhealthy woman only to experience a dead end of misery. Consider the ROI when choosing to place a lifetime commitment with any woman. Pay attention to red-flags, consider her character and choose according to what you really see not what you want.

The same would go for any place of business with shady dealings or any group that is not pursuing a path of strong ethic or purpose; that would not be a wise place to spend your valuable Commodity. Choose well.

While there are tons of words and concepts to describe what a Provider looks like, here are three of my most important aspects of a Provider.

Presence; Most men assume that the most valuable thing he can provide to his family is from earning money; a certain standard of living, shelter, food, ballet lessons (etc.), opportunities, fun stuff, or just stuff in general.

Most men just want their loved ones to experience a much better life than they had as a kid.

We will work hard and sacrifice personally to provide material goodness. Many men expect that is the expectation, to provide material stuff and good experiences. Some women expect this, a woman who thinks material things or a certain standard of living will bring her life is not the type of woman you want to choose. Most women and family members long for a man to provide something else as well, that is Presence.

Presence is the most important thing to provide. You can ask anyone about their experience with their father, what was your greatest memory or what did you long for the most. It will never be the stuff he provided from working so hard. It will always be the time we went fishing, or when he read books to me, or I wished he would have spent more time with me.

⟿ **Your kid doesn't give a shit about how much money you make.**

Providing the material things is essential for sure. But providing your being is most essential. YOU are the most important thing to provide to those you love. Your presence and just being there is prime and being there with intention is extraordinary. Knowing that you are absolutely important in the lives of those you love, helps you to create a great balance between your work and your presence.

As you grow in your capacities of presence; using your good voice, having positivity, engaging in play and adventure, attentiveness, setting boundaries and nurturing, you will begin to notice the how powerful your presence is in the lives of those around you.

Generous; A generous man is benevolent, a team player, brings essential needs, gives, advocates, is community oriented and makes a difference. He is kind-hearted, considerate and concerned for the well-being of others, especially those under his care. He takes care of needs and wants of those around him. He blesses others through his voice and thoughtful consideration.

This is where the choice of Commodities is lived out. For those I love and have chosen to commit to, I will generously give of all I have. I will be open and vulnerable with myself and my emotional heart. I will give of my time and freedom. I will engage in true and deep connection with good conversation and physical presence. I will be free with the goods I have earned and create good, fun, memorable experiences.

Most men are very generous, it is a deep part of our desire to provide. When there is a little appreciation, we will give of ourselves to the point of great personal sacrifice. All we need is consistent kindness, appreciation, enthusiastic sex and we are good to go. Throw in some consistent affection and most men are willing to give it all. Our hearts are not like Scrooge, we want everyone to thrive.

⤳ **A man who provides is generous.**

<u>Reliable;</u> As a concept of providing, reliability is when the people you have chosen to commit your energy to, have someone who they can trust. They can trust you to be there, to give your best and to handle things when they need to be taken care of.

A reliable man makes sure he is physically healthy. His self-care is strong and intentional, so he is thriving himself. He does this, so he is able to increase the capacity of his strength to achieve his own goals and to be reliable for others.

He is a hard worker, resourceful, creates solutions, problem solves, fixes things and makes things work. He is competent and persistent. He leads, has vision, makes plans, and makes decisions. He has ownership of his life and family, he engages in partnership and makes you so glad he is on your team.

He creates environments of safety and security. He strategizes ways to make sure everyone in his sphere of influence is doing well. He observes and pays attention to his surroundings and the well- being of others. He has what it takes.

Like a muscle, providing is one of those things you can exercise so it grows big and strong. The more you build your career, the more capable you are of providing a better lifestyle. The more you build your ability to be present, the more your relationships will be healthy and strong. The more generous you are with yourself, the closer you will be to others.

Even if you are a single man, you will have the opportunity to give, provide and supply goodness to people around you. As Provider, you have the opportunity to be on mission to change the world for good.

Other words to describe the Provider;

A Provider is also an advocate, skilled, capable, observant, loyal, committed, focus, self-care, on the move, influential, forward thinking, dependable, knows what needs to be done, count-on-able, physically healthy, hard worker, team player, resourceful, creates solutions, takes care of wants, leads, has vision, makes decisions, problem solves, fixes things, makes things work, competent, persistent, works hard, brings essential needs, nurtures, creates an environment of safety and security, ownership, partnership.

TLA

Each of the "Muscles" will have a TLA (**T**hree **L**etter **A**cronym) which gives an easy tool to remember the essence of what you will be developing with each particular Muscle. Hopefully this will help some of the content to be memorable.

The Provider TLA

BYC = Build Your Capital

Building Your Capital is an ever-increasing ability to make money, increase influence, build relationships and to expand your "kingdom". Do you remember how much you made per hour in your first job? I made 11 cents per tree yanking the new green growth (called suckers) from the inside of apple trees when I was 9 years old. Now I make a decent hourly wage as a therapist. My earning capacity has changed!

I have built my ability to make money over my life. I have earned two degrees, certifications and licenses to make that happen. I have gone through significant internships, supervision and training programs to build my skill. This provides us with the Power to make things happen in our own lives and in the lives of those we love. And with any person who would benefit from our generosity.

Our capital is also expressed in our influence and how we network or build the community around us. Having a strong network will provide some of the greatest help when you are in need or just a sense of connection and purpose. As a man of Power, Build Your Capital

The Protector Muscle

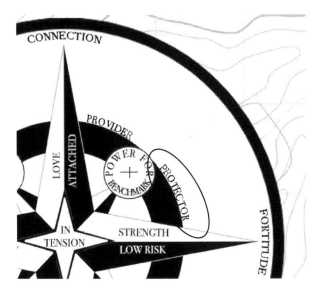

The Protector Muscle

In the Power For quadrant and leaning toward the side of Fortitude and Strength, the Protector Muscle is what it says; it's there for Protection. Protection exists for the care, well-being, safety and security of all in the Protector's sphere of influence. This is where it is still infused with Connection. It is using Power For to protect those you love and have chosen to be under your care.

Just as with your Provider Muscle, choosing the people you will protect in your life is very important. You need to use your best wisdom since protecting may very well cost you your life. Your protection is no small thing. Since it may include placing not just your well-being, but your life on the line potentially, regard it with those deep implications.

    ➴ **The desire to be a Provider and a Protector is deep within a man.**

All these decisions must be made with extreme sobriety. Do not choose a woman who lacks character. Do not go out and just rescue anyone who will not regard your well-being and care for your heart. This is one of the places of great foolishness for many men; choosing a woman who does not respect one of your greatest gifts; Protection.

Many men will choose a woman because she chooses you, because she likes you or because she is willing to have sex with you. This is just external validation for a man without a strong core, it feels good, but it is no reason to choose a woman.

Do not choose a woman who is unwilling to place herself under your care. This is part of the "submission" question in Christian circles. When it comes down to it, is your woman willing to submit to you? I am not talking about submitting to you as an authority who will tell her what to do. Does she respect you and is she also making an "all in" investment in your life together.? Does she trust you?

If a woman understands what being a Protector means, that you are willing to spend your Commodity with the ultimate price, then she will respect that in a way that shows she is willing to give fully in return as well. If a woman knows and respects this very significant gift, her posture will show it. If she doesn't respect this potential gift, don't give this type of woman the time of day. Find a woman who respects the fact that you are a Protector.

Comedian Bill Burr jokes that the idea that women make less than men is the way it should be. That there is a $1 hourly surcharge paid to men since in any emergency situation men will be required to protect, give up their seat in the lifeboat or make sure women and children are first. He thinks because of this, it is only right men make more per hour than women!

In reality, men have no problem being the protectors. We see it in every emergency, every shooting, every flood, men give it up. Men cover others and take bullets. Men gather their fishing boats and come to the rescue. It is what men do, without even thinking about it. Protecting is in our being.

One of the clearest ideas about men protecting is from the story from *American Sniper* that describes three types of people: wolves, sheep, and sheepdogs. Wolves are strong predators, they prey on sheep and anything that is weak or helpless. Sheep are oblivious, naïve and weak; they can get eaten by the wolves. Sheepdogs are strong and reliable, and they protect the sheep against the wolves. The challenge of the story is, "What kind of man will you be, son?"

Safety and security is the number one need of women. Men usually don't even have those on our radar. We must remember that "Safety is Job One!"

While there are tons of words and concepts to describe what a Protector looks like, here are three of my most important aspects of a Protector.

Vigilant; The Protector has his eyes open. He watches and is aware of surroundings. His vigilance is played out as there is just always something in the background of his mind, the commitment to make sure people are going to be safe under his watch.

Even though sometimes it is at the forefront of the mind, usually it is just under the surface, a passing thought about the nearest exit or a peculiar sound. Being vigilant is a way of being; observing self, others and surroundings. His intuitive is his best indicator. The "spidey sense" will give him the most valuable and timely information.

Vigilance is securing the perimeter. It is making sure everything is ok in our home. Remember the idea of Fortitude being a 'fort"? Securing the perimeter is having the fort secure. It is making sure everything is locked for the night. It is making sure the family is doing well.

While vigilance is surveillance and making sure of safety, it does not mean that there is no adventure. But while you are on an adventure with your kids camping or serving a meal downtown, you are on watch.

➔ Vigilance is usually just staying out of a mess.

One of the most difficult experiences for any man to process is when something happens under his watch, for instance, if a relative took advantage of one of his kids abusively or an accident happened during a fun event. These things happen, but when you didn't see it coming, it crushes something deep. The call is just to do your best.

It is deep within us to protect the innocence of children. We are heart-broken about stories of people who suffer abuse. Allow these stories to create motivation to be vigilant in your world, but not to keep you from play and adventure.

Prepared; A protector is ready, and he has taken precautions to have a strong perimeter. Depending on your neighborhood, you'll need to attend to your locks, windows and security. Is it wise to have firearms? What kind of protocol do we have with our police and fire house?

Am I ready physically? Am I out of shape? Many men prepare themselves by attending any type of martial arts class. Just about every strip mall has a hole-in-the-wall business with a class with Jiu Jitsu, Krav Maga, MMA, Karate, Boxing, Aikido, or other form of self-defense.

Learning to handle yourself physically is a huge way to be prepared. No one has any idea what may happen next in life. Being in good shape, knowing how to handle your body in a tussle, knowing how to navigate a conflict, just having a more confident posture is essential in being a Protector.

You may want to go through a concealed carry class, so you can legally carry a firearm with you wherever you go. Depending on your local laws and your own personal perspective, you can choose to do this or not. Regardless if you will carry or not, the class will provide some very valuable information to you.

There are classes on active shooter situations, how to handle conflict or how to keep your home safer. One of my favorite Bible ideas is the word "meek" from the phrase, "Blessed are the meek, for they shall inherit the earth." It does mean gentle and humble, but also a man who has great strength while being under control.

It is like a wild animal who is tame, but still holds its wild nature and ability to kill. It is being wild and fierce, but under control. I have heard it said that meek is one who has all the weapons but keeps them sheathed. It is keeping calm, even in the face of insults. Meek is not weak, but it is having great strength, and using that ferocity rarely, only when necessary, only when violence is the answer. Consider how prepared you are, because a Protector is prepared.

Sacrifice; Sacrifice is the willingness to give something up for something else, usually with a loss. Ultimately, it is about value. It may be my time. I value what I gain by giving my time to my work, so I can get something I value; a standard of living or some freedom. Every sacrifice is an exchange of one value for another.

I will sacrifice my life to save someone I love. I have said it before that most men would take a bullet without thinking to protect their family. There are things that are priceless, and my life is a fair trade. Whether it is time, freedom or your life, a Protector is willing to make sacrifices necessary to keep people they love from harm.

Choice again is a primary category here. Have I placed myself around people of such quality and love that I would not even question making ongoing and one-time sacrifices? Have I been wise with deciding who I would spend my Commodities with? How could I build a very healthy group or family of people around me that I would give so much of my life for?

Having deep connections creates some very deep meaning for men and that motivates the Protector.

Other words for Protector are;

A Protector is also described as intensity, aggressive, adversarial, defender, pathfinder, clears the way, a force to be reckoned with, trained well, willing to fight and wise not to, powerful, rescuer, deliverer, has your back, appropriately bad-ass, protects and begets innocence, force for good, fierce, spine, prepared to be violent, dangerous, risk-taking, bold, challenges, pursues, firm, defends the weak, seeks justice, fights for those who can't defend themselves, speaks against wrongs, ethic of justice, stands up, physical, mastery of physical being, intimidating, impenetrable, resilient, backbone, "not under my watch".

Protector TLA

BYP = Build Your Power

As the Provider is on an ever-increasing quest to increase his ability to build capital, the Protector desires to build his Power. This requires building a mind-set of vigilance, awareness, physicality, presence and even an understanding of violence. It is as though you will become your own Secret Service team for your family.

The Secret Service are the people called to protect important people like the president. They have training not just the ability to engage in physical altercation, but in the million ways to keep that from ever happening. They know how to see what is in the surroundings, what kind of postures people have, what seems suspicious, what looks normal. They intuitively know when to clear out before there is a need to engage.

➔ **Get the asset to the car!**

How would you begin to build your ability to become your own Secret Service? What could you do to be confident if you had to engage, but more confident in knowing your surroundings and when to clear out to keep everyone you love safe? Intentionally make a plan to increase your abilities and awareness. There are books and classes made just for this. Remember this is about becoming the strongest, most powerful man you can be so that you can love others well. Empower yourself!

Archetype; The Warrior

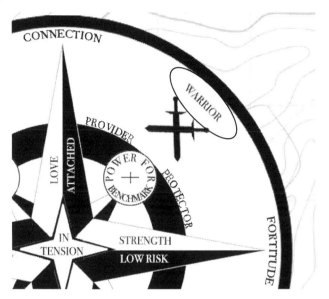

The Warrior Archetype

I will be presenting a central archetype for each quadrant. An archetype is something that is seen as an original pattern or model from which other new patterns are made. It would be like a copy of an original. The original is the archetype.

An archetype is the thing that came first, whether it is an idea, a type of person or a prototype of a human characteristic upon which all other humans are based. Carl Jung considered archetypes as an unconscious idea or pattern of thought or behavior which are inherited, carried on through generations and universally present in individual psyches.

Jung called it the Collective Unconscious; the archetype is the part of the psyche that is common to every culture in every era of history and mankind. The archetype is a pattern of behavior that is grounded in biology as instinct and is manifested in our actions. An archetype has developed as certain representations of those patterns in our cultural and personal stories which bring to life ideas and categories of our humanness.

These archetypes become enlivened within people as they encounter various experiences. As when you watch or read any story which follows the "Hero's Journey" categories. Books/movies like Star Wars, Lord of the Rings, Harry Potter or Avatar all have elements which seem to awaken our hearts to something deeper and exciting. Our lives are just normal, but something is alive inside of us that is piqued when we hear a good story or engage in an adventure.

There are many archetypes that have been identified; The King, The Warrior, The Sage, The Magician, The Trickster, The Lover, The Cowboy, The Everyman, The Queen, The Great Mother, The Hero, The Beauty, The Innocent, The Explorer, The Martyr, The Outlaw, The Creator, The Jester and The Poet/Warrior are some of the most mentioned.

As there are many, for this exercise I will use four main archetypes which will fit nicely into our map of masculinity. For the Quadrant of Power For, the archetype is The Warrior.

The Warrior coincides with the idea of Power, Strength and Fortitude. It comes alive in the world as being a Provider and a Protector. As well, the Warrior is always connected to his people. He is just not fighting a battle because he is just conflictual or contrary, he is fighting for the well-being of his people.

The Warrior wages war against chaos and entropy. The battle is against what can be called the "Outer Dragon". As things fall apart, he restores order, security and honor. This restoration requires a significant level of ferocity, aggression and intensity. In this category, his fight comes from without, not from within (that fight is in the next quadrant).

The Outer Dragon is a metaphor for all those things in life that bring harm, pain and chaos. We know we can never eliminate all threat, but the Warrior sets his heart to do the best he can for those he loves or for what he believes.

There are things in our world which destroy, steal and deceive. There are forces that thwart, there are those that are just malignant and there are those that are flat-out evil. The Warrior acknowledges that there is a battle to be fought in the physical realm, in the spiritual realm and in the realm of ideas. He engages to create safe and secure spaces for those he loves.

> ⮑ Evil brings challenge, you are forced to bring forth what you couldn't bring forth if you didn't have an adversary. The greater the thing you are to bring forth, the greater the challenge. - Jordan B. Peterson

The Warrior follows the motto of Power For; "I will become the strongest, most powerful man that I can be, so that I can care for and love others well."

This idea that a sense of being a Warrior is deeply rooted within the soul of every man as an archetype is part of our challenge if we have never experienced opportunities to be a Warrior.

We know something resonates in us when we hear a good story of a Warrior, so we know something is in us. We are drawn to competitions that have aggression or intensity, like MMA, Football, Hockey or Boxing. Why else did Fight Club intrigue a generation of men? Something is in us, that thing is the archetype of the Warrior.

So, this question comes up, "Would you rather be safe or strong?" The Warrior in us wants to be strong, to create safe for others. The Warrior wants to "kill it" at work so he can provide greatly. The Warrior wants to live to a higher code of honor to protect his flock. He is prepared, vigilant and ready.

The Warrior is "Meek" -He has the sword, but he keeps it sheathed. He is not combative nor pugnacious, he will do all he can to keep from a fight, but the Warrior is willing and able to engage when and only if it is necessary.

He knows that once you do engage, safety goes out the window for everybody, someone is going to get hurt. He will do all he can to retreat or escape a potentially dangerous situation, with humility and grace. Being able to not get in the situation in the first place is the best move. In the immortal words of Lynyrd Skynyrd, "Gimme three steps.", getting out of the situation is the next best move.

- Best move = stay out of the situation.
- Next best move = get out of the situation.

Getting down to business, is the worst and last move. When this happens, someone will get hurt and that is not a good option. Hopefully it will never get to that but be ready. Remember with your woman, safety is job one, so do your best to maintain safe environments.

Distortions of the Power For Quadrant

Every aspect of life seems to have a shadow or dark side. It is when any category of life lived out with immaturity or fear. We all have seen and experienced how power is abused. Here are three ways that this quadrant goes awry.

The first distortion is described as **"Power Over"** as a posture where strength is used to control, manipulate, intimidate and abuse. When the masculine is driven by fear or is attached to unhealthy outcomes, power is used in an abusive way "over" another person, which restricts their freedom, choice and personal power often resulting in violations and abuse.

Power Over is tyrannical; controlling and authoritarian. It is the corrupt politician, it is the playground bully, it is the controlling spouse and it is the manipulative boss. Each of these examples are based in fear and insecurity. People who take the Power Over posture are trying to control their environment to achieve something that will give them a sense of security or personal validation.

It is very difficult to navigate situations when people act this way. It feels as though all our power and freedom is gone. It is not, it just feels so. Our challenge is to commit that we will recognize it, stand up to it and never replicate it.

The second distortion is **"Powerlessness"** or a posture of chosen weakness or surrender. This posture occurs when masculine strength in essence is believed to be bad or even evil. Men will then choose to rebuke or repel any internal masculine strength that exists within in order to fit in, not cause harm or not be "that guy" who uses and abuses women.

The typical "Nice Guy" or SNAG (Sensitive New Age Guy) fits here. Many men are uncomfortable or even fearful of their own masculine strength. Even as you have read the previous pages you may have felt very uncomfortable as I outlined Fortitude and Power. Diminishing your strength is not healthy in any way. You've been designed to be a strong and powerful man, so take the challenge to grow in that even if it feels uncomfortable.

Often when men have a powerless posture, they move with passive aggressive or covert behavior. This is because they can't be overtly strong or forceful since that would break some kind of unwritten code or rule. Any movement from a powerless position looks weak and unmanly. It is never attractive to anyone. It just doesn't work well on any level.

Powerlessness is also seen as **"Unreliability"**. This is an aspect of the Provider Muscle. If a man lives in an "underfunctioning" way, that is he does not pull his own weight in any category, at home, work, on a team, or in a community. This often occurs when a man loses his heart or motivation because he has experienced some failure or received some input of unworthiness so he has chosen to give up.

A man who has chosen this path has lost hope that he will have any ability to bring change or to influence the world around him, he has taken on a "victim" posture. The loss of confidence will look like depression or sometimes abuse as he tries to make some kind of sense or reclaim some kind of power in a very unhealthy way.

These forms of the dark side of Power are deeply misinformed, quite immature and even repulsive to the true masculine soul. Take the time to begin to build Fortitude, Strength and Power For into your good heart.

Benchmark #1 Motto:

"I will become the strongest, most powerful man that I can be, so I can love others well."

Concrete Steps to Gain Power For:

Responsibility

> ➔ I am responsible for my life and I will engage in strong personal boundaries.

Understanding your own power means that you understand that you have agency in your life. You have choice and you are not a victim to what life throws at you. You understand that life is a beautiful dance with difficulties and victories all wrapped up in a spectacular package of growth and passion. As you grow in power, agency and responsibility you will begin to join the movements of how your Masculinity has been designed to influence in ways you never imagined. It will become fun.

Boundaries are lines, one side is ok or preferred behavior and the other side is not ok. It is very important to have good boundaries in your life. Speak up when you need to say no. Hold people accountable to treat you well, especially your woman. Stand up when you see evil or when things are not right. Make your presence known.

Self-Care

> ➔ To maintain personal strength, I must engage in intentional and consistent self-care.

Taking care of yourself is one of the most important things you can do to keep your power growing. Get in shape, get the sleep you need, eat well.

Get in to see your doc. Your check-ups with a doctor is a very vulnerable experience, you don't know what he is going to say. He may say you're good to go and keep up the good work, or he may have concerns about a possible cancerous lump. Get your butt in there.

Taking care of your body is huge, but care for everything else as well; your spiritual well-being and your relationships. Keep your spiritual heart alive and connected to your Source. Mend broken relationships and build your primary relationship. You'll be surprised how these parts of life help build your overall strength and influence.

Balance

⮞ Keeping a good balance in life will help me hold my power.

Be diligent to have margin and a good pace. Keep a good balance between Heart and Spine, be open yet keep your strength. Being the strongest most powerful man, you can be is exhilarating, and the balance is to use that strength for good, for the benefit of yourself and others. The balance between all the Cornerstones requires that you live in that tension.

Questions

Quadrant One is between the Low-Risk side of Fortitude and the attached side of Connection. It is becoming the strongest, most powerful man that I can be, so I can love others well. The Power For quadrant has the Muscles of Provider and Protector. It is built by developing the TLA's Build Your Capital (BYC) and Build Your Power (BYP). And it is lived out with the Archetype of the Warrior. What seems like the most important aspect for you to build?

The Power For Motto is "I will become the strongest, most powerful man that I can be, so I can love others well." This is about becoming a very empowered man. What comes to mind or how do you feel about using your energy and focus to become a very strong man?

The idea of using your Power For others rather than Over others is essential to living in mature Masculinity. In what ways have you experienced both of these forms of Power? What was it like and how did you respond?

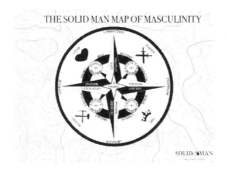

THE SOLID MAN MAP OF MASCULINITY

SOLID MAN

6 Quadrant Two – Solid Frame

Benchmark #2 – Solid Frame

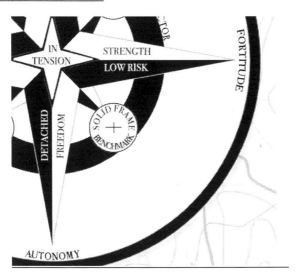

The Solid Frame Benchmark

At the corner between Fortitude and Autonomy is the Benchmark called "Solid Frame". Solid Frame is found where the Commodities of Strength and Freedom meet. Fortitude and Strength on one side with Autonomy and Freedom on the other. These categories seem to fit together like hand in glove and they create significant concepts for the life of a man.

107

Remember that the Fortitude/Strength side of the equation is where the concept of Power comes from. We have been designed to be powerful and strong. As the last quadrant was the interaction between strength and relationship, Benchmark #2 is about a man's relationship with himself, his autonomous self and his strength.

Solid Frame is the Benchmark in this quadrant. At the crossroad of Fortitude and Autonomy, it is having a strong self. It is internal Fortitude. Internal Fortitude that will withstand storms and hold up under pressure. It is developing a core that is immovable, sustainable and unshakable. Solid Frame is significant in that the Masculine has been designed to be driven and defined from deep internal realities found within the soul of a man. The Masculine has been designed to be solid in Freedom and Strength in a personal structure which is integrated, whole and internally referenced.

Solid Frame describes a state of confidence, concreteness and a sense of being grounded or unalterable. It is having clear boundaries because you know who you are, what you want and where you are going. It is having a solid internal core which is not driven by what other people think (not being a pleaser); but has an unalterable internal confidence and internal moral compass. Solid Frame describes a person with internal structure, stability, wholeness and consistency.

Solid is a word I have chosen as a primary word to describe manhood. If I were to only have one word to describe a healthy man, it would be the word Solid. Consider how a rock is Solid. It is firm, it has depth, it has gravity. The rock is there, usually to stay. You cannot easily move it. It is reliable, has substance and holds fast.

Consider how it is different than liquid. Anything Solid holds its own shape. The substance of its shape does not change except under the most extreme circumstances. It has stability and you know what it is when you see it and feel it. It is Solid.

Liquid has often been a word that describes how the Feminine moves. As the polarity of Masculine Solidness and Feminine Fluidity interact with each other there is attraction and bonding, much like poles on a magnet or molecular bonds in chemistry.

The Masculine has been described as a container for the Feminine. The container, being solid holds the shape and the fluid takes the shape of the container, whether it is a glass or a reservoir. As the Feminine energy is fluid, the Masculine can hold the energy in a way that allows for freedom and expression of the beauty of the feminine.

In a similar way the Masculine could also be described as the riverbanks and the Feminine the river itself. The riverbanks guide and lead the river to move in certain directions. The Feminine will push up against the banks, yet eventually move with the firmness of the riverbanks. Many women enjoy this artful dance, it is the designed movement between the masculine and feminine.

The energy of lightning is also a metaphor here as well. Imagine the Feminine being the lightning and the Masculine the lightning rod grounded into the earth. As grounded, the Masculine has the capability to direct the energy. This happens often in a relationship, much to the consternation of the one who is the lightning rod. If you are not grounded it is a horrible experience. If you are grounded, it is no problem directing the energy into a harmless direction. You don't have to carry it and you can stand up to it.

Being grounded is like being centered or anchored, also as an aspect of Solid Frame. Anchored or centered are terms which describe someone who is deeply connected to themselves and is somewhat immovable with their emotional or spiritual state of being. Having a strong internal frame of reference is how to develop a Solid core and to become anchored and centered in life.

Frame is a word that describes a basic structure that underlies something, like the foundation of a home. Usually it is something strong and firm that surrounds a picture or doorway. The Frame holds things all together. Framing is the part of building a house that is the basic structure of walls, headers, joists and rafters, it makes up the frame of the house.

The Frame of a man is his internal structure, which I often refer to as integrity. There is a design or blueprint that is intentional about the internal Frame of all men. The blueprint is what this map of Masculinity reveals. The first quadrant revealed the structure of Power-For, Protector and Provider. This quadrant is Solid Frame and the next two quadrants reveal even more of the blueprint and design of the structure of a man.

The word Frame is also used in the world of dance. With many ballroom types of dancing, the "lead" will hold frame with a strong posture, firm arms and confident movement guiding toward the next steps of the dance. Most women enjoy following a lead that has this kind of frame and are frustrated if there is no strong frame. This just happens to correlate almost precisely with real life.

As the second Benchmark of Masculinity, Solid Frame is an aspect that must be developed if you are going to become good at being a man.

Holding Frame in the face of any kind of difficulty or Void experience in life is not easy, but it is what we are shooting for. Sometimes men crumble as things get tough. If a wife criticizes it is met with immediate defensiveness. If a boss demands unethical behavior you do it out of fear of losing your job. If life gives you lemons, you go play video games or look at porn.

What is the thing that keeps a man solid like a rock? What will develop that internal Fortitude that holds fast under difficulty? What gives a man confidence enough to lead into uncharted waters? The answer to this was mostly answered in the Second Pillar, Embracing the Void. The Void is the place where we are initiated into confident manhood. We find out that we do have what it takes, and we are enough to handle just about anything that comes along.

Frame is concreteness and a sense of being immovable or unalterable. Frame is having clear vision because you know who you are, what you want and where you are going. This is not giving too much consideration to what other people think (not a pleaser), but having an unalterable internal confidence. Integrity is another word that describes this, integrity describes structure, stability, wholeness and internal consistency.

Solid Frame is something that is developed over time in our lives as we push ourselves into tough situations. It is grown when we stay in and embrace the Void for as long as is necessary. We often will intentionally engage in discomfort so we can grow. We find out who we are and what kind of stuff we are made of when we engage in uncomfortable situations and experiences.

- ᕙ **Find out what kind of material you are made of, push into discomfort.**

Men are made of some of the strongest materials you can imagine. Not only do we have good muscles, we have good hearts. We have strong abilities to build our intellect and logical processes. We have deep intuitive and instinctive strength. We are able to withstand incredible loss while maintaining firm control of a situation. Our souls are made of good identity and moral compass. We can take quite a bit.

Most of us have experienced good coaching. For me, the best coaches knew exactly how far he could push me. As a young man I had a very limited idea of what my body was capable of. I was pushed way beyond what I thought, and it produced some great outcomes for me in athletics.

What I am giving you here is the same thing. You are capable of withstanding so much more than you think. You have all the capability in yourself to become and be a man with incredible Solid Frame. You are way more than you have ever been told, you've got it all inside you.

This was what Pillar One was all about; creating a strong internal frame of reference. This quadrant of Masculinity is all about developing a strong internal integration of all your internal resources, a sense of wholeness and completeness and the strong internal frame and the confidence that it will hold fast in just about any circumstance.

> ☞ Solid Frame is fully expressed as a man is internally referenced, driven and defined by realities based in his true identity, his integrity, his intuition and his intention.

Solid Frame is not just a metaphor or an idea, it is a concrete reality which every man must seek. This is a significant way that a man becomes good at being a man.

> ☞ Remember this: "Masculinity is a deep reality present within the core of every man. It is revealed in a drive to be a generous and powerful force for good, founded upon a solid internal integrity and identity, expressed through purposeful and creative movement into the world, and lived out with passion for life and relationship."

The Muscles of Benchmark #2: Honor and Integrity

Reflecting the concept of Solid Frame, the two Solid Frame Muscles are Honor and Integrity. These Muscles are found between Fortitude and Autonomy and are expressed through the Commodities of Strength and Freedom.

The Honor Muscle

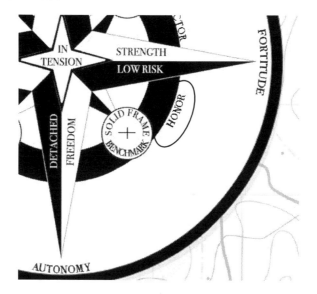

The Honor Muscle

In the Solid Frame quadrant and leaning toward the side of Fortitude and Strength is the Honor Muscle. Honor is an ancient virtue which speaks to deeply held internal beliefs and ways of seeing the world that seem archetypal or even sacred. Honor holds to standards set forth by ancient internal and communal realities.

Honor is worthy of respect and imitation. Honor is doing what's right, holding fast to one's own moral compass or code of ethic. Often a person of Honor has a "Code of Honor" that has a certain standard of conduct that they follow without hypocrisy.

They say there is no "honor among thieves", but that is not true, it's just a different code. Such as, you would never snitch. Everybody has some kind of belief system or worldview which guides how they move through life.

Everyone has a worldview or belief system, but does everyone have Honor? Not in the least, true Honor is based on some very basic principles. True Honor has ageless value; courage, benevolence, protection of the innocent, voice for the voiceless, value of all life, mercy, loyalty, consistency, character, hospitality, generosity and self-discipline are some of these values.

Honor is highly connected to two things, your name and your word. Your name is the character and substance of your identity behind your moniker (like Bob or Bill). Your name represents all that is under the surface of your being, expressed in your behavior, choices and movements in life. Many men will sell out their name without Honor, allowing lies or deceit to take them down. A man of Honor upholds his name with powerful self-respect. His name is one of his most valued possessions.

> ➴ "I have given you my soul; leave me my name!"   -
> John Proctor, *The Crucible*

A man's word is another priceless possession. As you cannot put toothpaste back in the tube, the words that come out of you are forever out there. A man of Honor will use his words and voice with generosity, grace, skill and blessing. He knows his words have deep meaning, especially to his children. He will speak with integrity and what he says is what he means. His words are words with Honor.

> ➴ "Be impeccable with your word"
> 1st of *Four Agreements* – Miguel Ruiz

Many groups throughout history have had a Code of Honor. The Samurai of Japan had the Bushido Code, there was the Medieval Code for the knights across Europe, many warrior cultures like the Spartans had a Warrior Code which guided behavior. Even today there are codes of Honor in our armed services which outline the highest values. Living with Honor is living with expression of the highest values of humanity.

Here are a few values that I have chosen for you to develop as you begin to exercise your muscle of Honor;

Justice; Justice is what is right, good and noble. It is a form of fairness, that each person would be treated rightly under the law with the same consequence.

Whether it is a contract determined by mutual consent of a group, rules determined by the natural state of being or laws given by God, justice is a set of rules or laws which determine right behavior in community.

As a man of Honor, you uphold justice in all circumstances. You will fight for the rights of people who are abused and dispossessed. You will stand for ideals which you know are right and honorable. It is within the quote; "I will defend your right to disagree with me to the death." As an internally referenced man you will have a set of core beliefs that will guide you through life. Standing for these in the defense of others is justice.

Much has been said that good people have been led astray to do despicable acts (as in Nazi Germany) when they lived for external ideals rather than internal value and truth (justice). They thought they were fighting for justice but had lost their internal Frame. This external pressure to belong or fit in to something greater, along with the strong narratives given, has deceived many people to do horrible things in our history.

We would like to believe that we would stand if ever those moments came to us, even to the point of death. But if our Frame of justice is fragile in any way, we too could fall to this kind of tyranny. When/if our "Give me liberty or give me death" moment ever comes, may we be found to have a strong Frame of justice.

Authority; Similar to dominion and dominate, the word authority is somewhat reviled in our world today. Authority is power, ability to make decisions and to have control. Authority as power reminds us of the Power-For construct. Real authority begins with having a strong internal authority. Within myself, I have power, ability to make decisions and self-control. Ultimately you can only control yourself.

When authority is the tyrannical or Power-Over type of power, it is unhealthy and used wrongly. As a man grows into a person with deep internal authority, his influence increases greatly. People are willing to follow since they know his authority is set to empower and release others to live well. This is the true authority that a man with Honor wields.

Becoming a man of authority is a great goal in life. To have good, positive influence in the lives of those you love and in your community is a significant goal. To lead others toward increased well-being, confidence and freedom is true authority.

<u>Responsibility/Ownership</u>; Many people live with the posture of victim, where they have no interest in agency or responsibility in life. They are being "done to". Masculinity is the opposite, it has a strong sense of agency where responsibility is taken for just about everything. Being responsible creates a posture of power and authority. Responsibility places you in a position of capability and competence to get the things done that you want to get done. Instead of being "done to" you are "doing" the world.

> ➔ **Responsibility is the meaning of life, pick something up and carry it!   - Dr. Jordan B. Peterson**

Often men are reluctant to take responsibility since they will be blamed for mistakes or when things go wrong. You know, it is always the man's fault. While this seems unjust, it is just fine, since this places you in a position of power and volition. Would you rather have power or be a powerless victim? Take "The buck stops here!" mentality. No longer being the victim, you will begin to have real control over your own life. This is a strong aspect of Honor.

<u>Fidelity</u>; Fidelity is faithfulness to something. It is fully giving your heart and loyalty to a cause or a person. It is a commitment to that cause or person's well-being and success. Fidelity is a strong byproduct of having a Solid Frame and is a very clear part of what it means to have Honor. For a man of Solid Frame, his Fidelity does not easily waver.

<u>Conviction</u>; Conviction takes belief to a higher level. I not only believe some thing but it is a deep sense that that some thing is right, or it is the right way to do or to be. A man with conviction holds fast to this sense with an uncanny focus which sometimes even feels over the top, especially if there is some evidence to the contrary. Like Fidelity, Conviction does not waver, it remains secure and locked in.

<u>Character</u>; A man's Character is his deep moral, ethical and personal qualities. It is the inherent defining aspects of who a man is. In this sense it is just not that he has a personality or personal qualities, but he has a sense of self that is quality. His being has an immovable grouping of qualities that are the essence of a good, masculine man. He is someone people will look up to as he moves through life.

Other Words to Describe Honor

Honor is also described as standing up, standing firm, setting boundaries, unapologetic, speaking clearly, holding fast, non-argumentative, not pugnacious, self-controlled, honorable, endurance, resilient, prepared, vigilant, responsible, goodness, self-controlled, physically present, intentional, virtuous, temperance, open, insightful, doesn't worry, doesn't wallow, is present, holds strong in fear, decision maker, ethical, unwavering, truthful, aware, self-confronts, confesses, admits wrongs, honest, sure, anchored, impeccable with his word, uncompromising, centered, internal moral compass, wise, aware of sacred, humility, gratitude, values, stability, faithful, unwavering, grounded, and spiritually connected.

Honor TLA

IWD = Impeccable in Word and Deed

As with all aspects of the Map of Masculinity, true Honor is lived out from an internal frame of reference. Having a strong goal to be impeccable in both your words and your deeds is important. Impeccable means that you are upholding the highest standards of propriety. This means your word is true, in all you say. This means that your deeds are honorable in all you do.

This simple way to live out Honor gives a man the ability to have great influence as he strengthens his voice and presence in any situation by keeping a firm grasp of his deep internal truths. He will build trust more readily, he will be more reliable and anyone on his team (whether family, work or sports) will be able to count on him.

The Integrity Muscle

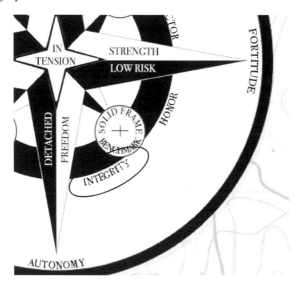

The Integrity Muscle

In the Solid Frame quadrant and leaning toward the side of Autonomy and Freedom, you will find the Integrity Muscle. For this muscle to really become yours you must remember that there are three main aspects of Integrity.

The first is that Integrity is about developing an internal structure, like a building with "structural integrity" will not collapse even under extreme conditions. Your solid, immovable internal structure is your goal as you build this muscle.

Secondly, Integrity is about developing integration, in which a system or a person lives in a holistic way. Integration brings all parts of a man into complete working order. Many have lost the ability to integrate important parts of ourselves, like emotions, wisdom, mind, body and spiritual aspects of life; therefore, we have lost our integrity, often. Because of shame, we have been dis-integrated and we are unable to live in an integrated way.

And thirdly, Integrity is about developing wholeness, like an integer. A whole number is complete, lacking in nothing. A solid man of integrity is whole and complete. Other people in his life are necessary for a full life of thriving, but he is solid in wholeness, there is no "You complete me" BS.

Building Integrity in your life is a lifelong endeavor. You will always have room to grow. As you develop this deep internal core, you will build so many strong parts of you and your confidence will soar. You will develop the Solid Frame. Integrity has the internal structure, the integration of all your good parts and wholeness. Here are a few other concepts that will help you learn how integrity is part of your life.

Wise; The man of integrity is constantly on a search for wisdom. Remember that wisdom is optimum judgement with optimum action. It is using the best information to make the best move in life. Integrity not only has wisdom as its goal, wisdom is the essence of integrity at its core. The integration of the internal resources within the frame of a man is one of the most profound avenues of discovering wisdom.

Wisdom is also found with accumulating knowledge and understanding through collecting ideas and beliefs from scriptures, great literature, wise people and history. If he does not know the answer or needs more information, he will ask questions to increase his knowledge base, even for directions! He will ask for help with humility. Because he gathers all this good intel, a man with Solid Frame has a deep well of wisdom within his Frame.

Compass; A man with Integrity can be trusted to be a light in a dark world and a guide in the midst of uncertainty and chaos. He may not know exactly where to go or what to do, but he has the internal tools to make the best move with the information available. With his Integrity he has a good sense of "True North" and is oriented to be able to discern which way is the right way. He able to guide and lead well in most situations.

Confident; The man of Integrity is confident in his inner capabilities. He knows he can handle just about any situation that may come his way. He is aware that his internal resources will guide him well. He is well practiced in listening to his intuition, spirit and emotional processes, and knows these have guided him beautifully in the past.

His posture is strong, sure and upright. He is not a poser and has left the feeling of being a fraud behind long ago, since he now knows who he is and what he is capable of. His confidence is real and not contrived. It is not arrogant or boastful. It is a quiet, sure sense that he has what it takes and that nothing needs to be proven or acknowledged.

Grounded; This man is anchored and grounded into something deep and strong. Not only does he have confidence that he can handle just about any situation that may arise, his being is locked into the depth of the foundations of life itself. As part of something much larger than himself, he anchors spiritually to his Source and physically to the Earth. He is connected. Because of this deep connection to self and to Source, he will maintain Frame as he moves through life in situations that used to crumble him.

Other Words to Describe Integrity;

Integrity is also unshakable, integrated, whole, complete, structure, internally referenced: internally defined identity, internally driven, true self, well-defined, real, authentic, knows who he is and what he wants, unattached, indifferent, differentiated, conscious, deep awareness of internal realities, resourceful, emotionally aware, physically aware, relationally aware, introspective, non-judgmental observer, and disciplined.

Integrity TLA

HTC = Hold The Center

Holding the center comes from an idea from the poem by W.B. Yeats, *The Second Coming.* One line in the poem says this, "Things fall apart; the centre cannot hold;" referring to the cultural state of things in post-World War One Europe. For our endeavor, I do not have such a bleak outlook. I believe men can "Hold The Center" in great times and in the most difficult times.

Holding the Center has less to do with the external realities of our culture (keeping the machine running), but the maintaining a strong sense of self in a deep internal place. If men are able to Hold The Center internally, there will be positive ramifications in marriages, families, communities and eventually the entire world. When things do fall apart (either in society or in a family), which they will, the center will hold when individual men keep their own centers held.

If a significant number of men were able to Hold their internal Center, in any circumstance, the world would always come out stronger and evil would not win as often. All it takes is for a few men to speak up, to stand up and to be willing to hold against evil or entropy which then will change the course of our communities, our world and history itself.

Solid Frame Archetype; The King

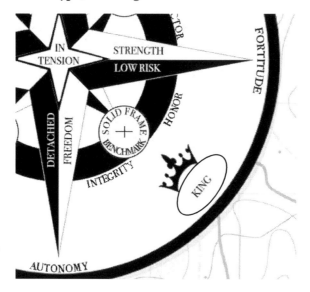

The King Archetype

Many images come to mind when you consider the word "king"; you may think of obese Henry the 8th with purple robes and rings, King John the Crusader, King Arthur and the Knights of the Roundtable, King David, King Solomon or King Herod from the Bible, Screwy King Louie from Jungle Book or the multitude of characters vying for the Iron Throne in the Game of Thrones. Whoever comes to mind there are characteristics that qualify that individual to be a king.

A king is a ruler who has authority and sovereignty over a place or group of people. It is usually a position given by birthright or taken by force. Regardless, the man sitting in the throne now has control and power that no one else has. He has the power to dictate the direction of the country, what people will do, and the laws that determine behavior of his subjects.

In the Solid Frame quadrant, the Archetype of King is about being a man who has control and sovereignty over his kingdom. For most of us this idea feels like a stretch or pushing into something uncomfortable. Especially as Americans who for our entire lives have been taught that kings are something that would cause a good ol' revolution. We have fought for our independence and by God, we will keep it. To which I say, of course, now that you have sovereignty over your own life, be the king of your own life.

Sovereignty is independence or self-governance. It is expressed as freedom to be and do as you want. The Western ideals of individual freedom were developed from two arenas, Greek Intellectualism and Christianity. Both of these forms of thought and belief placed a significant level of importance in personal or individual sovereignty. Each person was able to develop their own freedom and self-governance.

Consider your life, it is your kingdom. Your life is your playground. It is the space upon which you build what you want and desire. You see the great works of men who have come before you; Infrastructure, Inventions, Ideas. These men have created and developed kingdoms.

In comparison, we often see ourselves as small, meaningless or powerless, "I am not a kingdom builder", you say to yourself, "I don't have a kingdom". This is where you are so wrong. You have a kingdom. Even if right now it is small, in the smallest form your kingdom is you. And with all the abundance our world offers, your kingdom will grow mighty if you have vision and intention to build it.

Consider this, we experience so much more luxury than any king in all the fairy tales or real history ever did. They did not have plumbing (toilets, running water, hot showers), electricity (lighting, appliances, tools, tech), transportation (trains, planes, automobiles), food (stocked shelves, year-round seasonal food, restaurants) or communication (phone, texting, email, wifi, interwebs). Today, even the poorest of Americans live in more luxury than Solomon, Cinderella, Henry VIII or Charlemagne.

Our kingdom is made of all the services that are available to us at our whim; Amazon products, coffee, gas stations, delivery, medical/dental services, a flight this weekend to Las Vegas or just the ability to call home. Think of all your servants at your disposal who move into your service anytime you want something. You have a kingdom. We are all kings with luxury beyond anything a king of old could even imagine.

You have all that you need, life is abundant. Your woman is your queen, enjoying all this by your side. You can create a relationship you desire; you can build her up into the beauty as she has been designed, or you can break her down. You have that kind of power. You can build your kingdom to reflect goodness, beauty and justice, or you can let it be small with anger, addictions and revenge.

Whether or not you would follow the Bible, it speaks to the idea that the man is designed to be the leader of the household, like I am saying, the King. In the Bible the Apostle Paul talks about how the man is the "Head" of the wife in a similar way that Christ is the head of the man and the church. This is not a command or something to obey, but a reality of life, something that is, something that is internal.

- ➔ But I want you to realize that the head of every man is Christ, and the head of the woman is man, and the head of Christ is God. - First Corinthians 11:3

- ➔ For the husband is the head of the wife as Christ is the head of the church, his body, of which he is the Savior. - Ephesians 5:23

Men have found themselves in a position where their woman will "let" them lead or give them permission to make decisions. This is so backward to how things have been designed as though the woman is the head. The idea of being the "head" is what I am talking about being the King. Don't wait, don't ask, just BE what you have been designed to be.

- ➔ **Don't wait for permission. Be the King!**

It is time to blow the hell out of the small kingdom you have had and rebuild it into abundance and greatness. Take your queen, your space, your life and create a great vision for what you want and what will make you come alive, then begin to build your great kingdom. Expand into this great world with intent and love.

Own your own life and your own story, rewrite the narrative and create a beautiful ending. You have everything you need to do make it so. As a man with Solid Frame you are a King!

As a guardian of your realm, you have a sphere of influence no matter how small or large. It starts with you and then extends to your family, workplace, friends, and your community. You have the potential for more influence than you ever realized.

The King is centered. As centered, he has a strong connection with his Source or the transcendent. Even the king is under the power and influence of God. When a king considers himself as greater than the transcendent, his hubris overtakes him, and his kingdom fails.

A King is decisive. He is able to choose and make decisions based on the wisdom he has collected internally throughout his life. He considers the well-being of his subjects (wife, kids, employees, etc.) and makes choices for the best of all in his kingdom.

A King is integrated. As a man with Solid Frame, he trusts his internal processes and moves with confidence and strength. Since he is well on his journey to slay the Dragon within, he pursues the Dragon without. He creates order out of chaos and expands integration from within to without.

> ⤏ "The King has not only integrated all the other archetypes but seeks this wholeness in other areas of his life as well. He mends broken relationships, keeps his word, acts with honesty, and takes responsibility for his actions. He is who he says he is; he doesn't have one set of principles for Sundays and one for the rest of the week." – Brett McKay, Art of Manliness

The King inspires others to greatness, blessing all under his care to do well and to experience abundance. He recognizes and honors others for who they are, what they have achieved, and he sees greatness in others continually moving them towards even more greatness. As his power grows, so does the power of all around him.

The King leaves a Legacy; he has a deep desire to leave the world in a much better place than when he arrived, this is an essential aspect of the King Archetype. He carries his power with the Power-For posture, where he is dominant, but not dominating. He is an influential leader, leading to the Promised Land.

Distortions of the Solid Frame Quadrant

The two main distortions of the Solid Frame quadrant to watch out for are **Spinelessness** and **Lack of Leadership**.

Spinelessness is having a very weak frame, it is when a man is Externally Referenced, and he lives by the expectations of others or doing what would make others pleased with him. A person is externally referenced when their identity and/or their motivations are determined by what external influencers think or expect of them. When categories external to you define or drive you, a man will lose his Integrity.

When Solid Frame is lost he is no longer driving his own life from an internal reference using the vast resources which exist within. An externally referenced individual is the raft on the ocean, driven by the wind and current without determination or control over his own life. The negative consequences of such a life are numerous and profound.

Because his life is about pleasing others or living up to their expectations, he has no backbone; he does not stand up for what is right nor does he stand straight with a posture of confidence.

He is also Spineless because he lives in compartmentalization which is the propensity to live from segmented categories in life. Some people will describe this as having different "rooms" in your house of life. Each room will have a separate set of values, identity, expectations or other variables. This is the life of a Chameleon, living in diverse ways in distinct parts of life; work, school, home, etc. Personal Integrity and the Integrated Self is lost completely, and the self is dis-integrated into parts with no solid structure or wholeness. Therefore, he will not hold fast to his values or moral compass.

The Spineless man also lives in Secrecy, which is another result of the non-integrated self which is externally based on toxic-shame. The life of secrecy places the individual into a position of isolation/aloneness or hiddenness where several various "fig leaves" need to be worn to keep the illusion of wholeness or value. Since he hides significant parts of himself, he will never be able to stand tall when the spine is called upon.

Lack of Leadership occurs when a man fails to understand his masculine soul, his role in family or community and his own ability to create the life he wants. He allows others to guide and direct his own life and direction. Leadership is influence where a man will guide and direct not only his own life, but the lives of the ones he loves and cares for in a way that takes deep consideration for the well-being of them.

The man with no leadership allows other forces or people to take the reins. Leadership requires that you know who you are and what you want. That is how leadership is done. If you do not know what you want and where you want to go, you will never lead your own life nevertheless anyone else's. This man has no vision for what he wants, therefore he has no influence.

Surprisingly this is where abusive men are developed. Since they have no power to direct their own lives they think their only option is to be aggressive or controlling to get what they think they need.

Benchmark #2 Motto:

"I know who I am and what I am capable of, I will influence my world from a Solid Internal Frame with honor and integrity; things will fall apart, but my Solid Frame will hold fast, my center will hold."

Concrete Steps to Gain Solid Frame:

Responsibility

> ◑ I am responsible for my life and I will engage in strong personal boundaries.

Gaining ownership in the area of Solid Frame requires that you actually start to have Solid Frame. You must begin to see yourself as responsible for your life, you are not a victim, or even an active participant in your own life. You must take full responsibility for your own life and take it where you want it to go.

First, begin to notice how you ask permission, say you are sorry, hesitate or second guess yourself. These are all ways we live in someone else's frame. Just take time to notice, don't kick yourself for it, just see it for what it is.

Secondly, start to choose to do things in small areas of your life; go golfing, go out to beer with friend, or choose to go workout. Live in your own frame.

Thirdly, lead your own life. This is yours, no one else's. Take ownership and run with it. Trust your internal resources and make those good healthy wise choices.

Self-Care

> ◑ To maintain personal integrity, I must engage in intentional and consistent self-care.

The King must care for himself, so he can move with strength, intent and wisdom in his kingdom. If you don't listen to your internal resources, you will not live to your fullest. Trust your body, listen to wisdom about caring for your body and then implement those things.

Taking care of yourself is how you will maintain Solid Frame. Just like building your power, get in shape, get the sleep you need, eat well and get the medical help you need, especially if you're not sleeping well. This is the most internally referenced quadrant, so listen carefully to your internals and choose wise actions accordingly to keep care of your most valuable resource, you.

Balance

> ◑ Keeping a good balance in life will help me hold my center.

This quadrant is quite strong on the side of internal fortitude. Living with internal fortitude is like being a solid rock that doesn't move. Be that rock. Your balance will be developing proficiency in the other quadrants while being the immovable stone. This is part of where the paradoxes become real, each quadrant seems mutually exclusive of the others. Maintaining balance between all these concepts will be a huge part of mastering this process of becoming good at being a man.

Now we will move from building your own inner kingdom to expanding your world and your outer experience as we develop quadrant three.

Questions

Quadrant Two is at the crossroads of Fortitude and Autonomy, where we develop an incredibly strong internal sense of Fortitude. The motto is; "I know who I am and what I am capable of, I will influence my world from a Solid Internal Frame with Honor and Integrity; things will fall apart, but my Solid Frame will hold fast, my center will hold." It has the Muscles of Honor and Integrity, The TLA's of Impeccable in Word and Deed (IWD) and Hold The Center (HTC) and the Archetype of King.

What seems like the most important aspect for you to build?

Balancing Fortitude (being strong and closed) and Autonomy (standing on your own two feet) can be a challenge to some who have not developed a solid sense of self and differentiated identity, how have you been stuck with either needing others to validate you (not a strong self) or unwilling to embrace being strong?

Solid Frame means you have an internal structure that is immovable and firm. In what ways is that true for you and how it's not true for you?

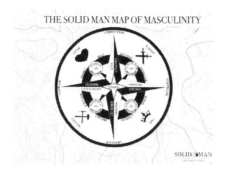

THE SOLID MAN MAP OF MASCULINITY

7 Quadrant Three - Expansive

Benchmark #3 Expansive

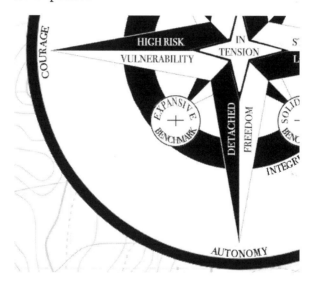

The Expansive Benchmark

At the corner between Autonomy and Courage is the Benchmark called "Expansive". Expansive is found where the commodities of Freedom and Vulnerability meet. Autonomy and Freedom on one side and Courage with Vulnerability on the other. At first glance this does not seem to fit into the masculine life, this is because we have been taught that Vulnerability is verboten to men. Nothing could be further from the truth and the concept of Expansive will show this.

A man experiences Freedom in this quadrant in that he moves with intention into his world. This is about Courage in that this free movement and action requires facing uncertain outcomes and fearful possibilities with Courage. The term I use here is Expansive.

Expansive means that a man is active, empowered, free. His presence is Expansive; moving and growing as he makes a positive difference and influencing with purpose. He moves into his world, by penetrating and creating life with his presence, voice and strength. The people around him experience an active, decisive and influential force, his life experience expands into the world and his influence grows.

⮕ **An Expansive man is a man with Direction.**

Although he will enter restful moments, you will often find the expansive man moving into, going toward, pursuing and actively creating things with freedom and intent. Even though he engages intentionally with domestic aspects of life, he is not domesticated and maintains a certain untamed wildness. He often desires adventure and the unknown. He loves variety and imagination.

His life is continually expanding into greater presence and influence. He creates a life of thriving for himself and those around him. This aspect of Masculinity "does", it is not comfortable with being "done to". Being active and initiating action and making things happen is what it means to be "doing" life. Sitting back, passively watching life go by and allowing things to happen without any influence does not fit the Expansive masculine soul.

⮕ **80% of life is just showing up. - Woody Allen**

Expansive means to grow, move into, penetrate, or to build influence. This is actually how a man's body has been designed. Our penis represents this metaphor well. It is designed to grow bigger and harder, and then penetrating into an empty space, all while planting seeds of life. So it is with a man's life.

Expansive means to create something out of nothing. Where there was only potential or sometimes even nothing, his influence of courageously entering into the Void and creating something is an act of godlike creativity.

This requires great Courage and Vulnerability since you are entering into the unknown or uncertainty (the Void). There is no proof of any positive outcome, only the desire to make something great happen. Initially, a man will have no proof if he has what it takes or if he will measure up, but confidence follows courage.

These great unsettled questions show that the endeavor to be Expansive requires Courage to even start. This is why many men sit on the sidelines, neglecting this powerful part of their souls. They are fearful that they may be found out to be a fraud or a poser, which incidentally is highly unlikely if they give it a go.

> ☞ My life expands or contracts in direct proportion to my courage. - Tim Ferriss

Men desire to give the fullness of their personal gifts to all who are around them, which creates a deep legacy that will exist long after they are gone. Creating a different life for loved ones is a profound passion for most men, as we talked in Quadrant #1 with the Provider and the Protector. Along with creating spaces of safety and well-being, men also look outward with vision of something more.

This vision for something more may be for family or community, but often it is just for him. It is for him, because he desires to go into, to penetrate, to see or to experience life to the fullest. Often, we will mock a young man's desire to jump off a cliff in Switzerland in a wingsuit, but we will still be in awe of the video that comes out on Youtube.

But it is just not jumping off a cliff, it is also doing deep scientific research toward sub-atomic places, developing new technology from crazy ideas or considering exploration of the stars. It is entering into the wilderness and seeing things few have seen or pursuing wildlife. It is gaining proficiency in relationships by hiring a relationship coach or reading books or listening to podcasts because you want to grow in your relational influence. It is creating a business or a new way to do anything.

In his essence a man has a deep desire to move into, to discover and to experience. This is what it means to be Expansive, to take his autonomous self and with Courage and Vulnerability move into spaces he has not yet explored. From these experiences, his life will expand, his confidence will expand, his self-image will expand, his relationships will expand, and his influence will expand. He will become a bigger person.

Expansiveness moves a man into discomfort and discomfort exposes us to what we fear the most. And this in turn grows us up into maturity and develops mastery in our lives. There is no other way to grow or to expand. You must embrace your deepest fears and expose yourself to the things that have haunted you your entire life.

☞ **The size of your problems is the size of your life.**
Zan Perrion

Rather than avoid and escape when faced with uncomfortable experiences, the Expansive life moves into those times with Courage and faces them head-on. This is where you live life and where you grow.

The Expansive life is a life which engages in Vulnerability in that you choose to put yourself into situations which will stretch you toward personal growth and increasing influence. You will never be Expansive without exposing yourself to situations which create discomfort or represent your deepest fears, like possible rejection, intimate or difficult conversations, potential conflict, increasing the tension, keeping an open heart, speaking from your heart or exposing yourself to things that you fear like heights or rejection.

Remember that Vulnerability is High Risk. It takes Courage to be Vulnerable and Vulnerability is required as you move into open, uncertain spaces. As you do this you will continually expand your personal capabilities and influence.

Expansive means that a man is active, empowered, free and influencing with purpose, penetrating and moving into his world, creating the life he wants and moving with intent with the people around him.

Expansive is epic. It is the great journey of the hero, of the entrepreneur or the explorer. Most importantly it's the journey of every man who desires to be a man. Expansive describes the greatest stories we have heard; it is Quiqueg experiencing the madness of Ahab, it is Frodo climbing Mt. Doom, it is Jesus facing death for mankind. You can think of your favorite stories, fiction and non-fiction, they all are expansive and epic, going way beyond the "normal" life. This is the Hero's Journey.

Expansive describes every small choice each man makes, essentially because it is a choice. Choice is the movement out into the world and into action. Even if it is the choice to get out of bed or to shave, it is a choice. Choice makes you into a creator and not a victim. Choice comes from our agency and being a person with responsibility and ownership. You can choose to sit, or you can choose to stand. What will it be? Each small choice is where Expansive thrives, or dies.

The Muscles of Benchmark #3: Explorer and Initiator

Reflecting the concept of Expansive, the two Expansive Muscles are the Explorer and the Initiator. These Muscles are found between Autonomy and Courage and are expressed through the Commodities of Freedom and Vulnerability.

The Explorer Muscle

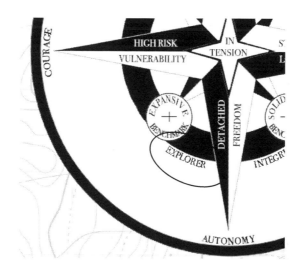

The Explorer Muscle

In the Expansive quadrant and leaning toward the side of Autonomy and Freedom is the Explorer Muscle. Exploring has been a significant aspect of the lives of men from the beginning of time. It is an ancient calling which speaks to a deep sense of needing to see the world or anything that has not been seen yet.

As you have read history, you may have been enthralled with some of the earliest explorers; Marco Polo, Leif Erikson, Neil Armstrong, Ernest Shackleton, just to name a few adventurers. Those who have left home to chart new territory, open new lines of trade or go where no man has gone before hold a dear place in our lives and history. There is something that resonates and connects with us when we remember these great people.

But there is even more to exploring than discovering new lands. Some of the greatest explorers were inventors or writers or mathematicians or engineers. Scientists and researchers are exploring constantly. Just because Thomas Edison did not leave his lab, does not mean he did not do incredible exploration.

Consider the quest to understand the world at the atomic or quantum levels. The dive into the smallest "nano" thing is exploration at its finest. Just as considering the stars, nebulas and galaxies is explorations on a grand scale, looking into the smallest world is exploration as well.

Exploring could be exploring inward realities. For you personally as you read the Solid Man materials you are on an exploration for the truth about your soul. It is a quest. It is exploring what you are made of and who you truly are. Self-discovery is also a very considerable aspect of the Explorer.

Part of your quest could be Exploring deeper into your relationships and how you came to be living like you are. Thinking about your family of origin or various choices you made in life are all part of your personal exploration. It could be an intentional pursuit of your woman, finding the nuances of who she is and how she thinks and what she needs.

Exercising this muscle could be traveling or visiting new places. It could be going into the wilderness hunting, hiking or fishing. It could be finding new places to eat or new beers or wine. It could be finding new way to do things or places to run. It could be exploring with different ways to have sex or to kiss.

It could be taking up a new thing to master like a musical instrument or martial art. It could be finding that very cool artist that really fits your style. Or going to a new part of town that you've never been. Or building a relationship with a culture you have never encountered. An entrepreneur is on a continual exploration of discovering new avenues of influence in business or way to create wealth or generosity.

There are a million ways to expand your Explorer muscle, but only two things are really required; 1) curiosity and 2) get your butt out there!

Here are some more ways that the Explorer is defined.

Penetrating; As I said earlier, our physical being is quite the metaphor for how a man actually is designed to move into his world and plant seeds of life!

In this way the Explorer moves into, enters, takes his presence into his world, enjoys the pleasure of moving into, brings life, reaches out, pursues, life-giving, pushes through, appropriately forceful, breaks new ground, sexually competent and responsible. I know this is somewhat risqué, but it is a significant way a man makes a difference in his world.

Adventurous; The Explorer faces fear, leans into uncertainty, finds new paths, looks for new frontiers, is ready for anything, prepared, pushes into risk, is appropriately risky, is equipped for the journey, he embraces mystery and the unknown, and has a strong sense of the sacred or aspects of life that have deep and profound meaning. He knows his life is a journey in which he will never make the destination, so he will find enjoyment and pleasure in the process of discovery and experience.

Magnanimity; Joseph Pieper says that, "Magnanimity is the expansion of the spirit toward great things; one who expects great things of himself and makes himself worthy of it is magnanimous." The Explorer is magnanimous as he allows his spirit and influence to expand into life. His presence grows day by day, eventually becoming a blessing to all who know him. His personal generosity of spirit and joy is like a good virus in his community which brings confidence and empowerment to all.

Play; I think that Dr. Brené Brown defines play accurately when she says that "play is doing something where you lose track of time." This means you could be doing anything, a game, a project, a conversation, exercising, reading, whatever. It is play if you are enjoying yourself so much that you are not aware of time or how much time has elapsed. The Explorer often is engaging in activities that is play. Even if it is working or doing something that takes great effort, it is play. Play with an element of danger or risk is central to being the Explorer.

Other Words Describing the Explorer

The Explorer by nature is also curious, inquisitive, intentional, he moves into, he pursues, he embraces mystery and the sacred, humorous, fun, he gets out there, travels, courageous, daring, bold, playful, man of action, spatially aware and free.

The Explorer TLA

PTV = Penetrate The Void

I have spoken much of the Void in Pillar Two. The Void is that place of Uncertainty, Emptiness, Limitation and Death. It is that space where there is nothing, the unknown or mystery. Mastering your Masculinity depends on your willingness to allow the Void to become a good friend as you embrace it regularly. Remember, that Void creates confident men.

Penetration is the act of moving into something, sometimes even forcefully. It has the obvious sexual connotation, as a penis would penetrate a vagina, an apt metaphor, but it is so much more. The Explorer seeks to penetrate the world or life in general, by moving into it with intention, vigor and playfulness. He seeks to discover and see what there is to see.

He seeks to experience all there is to experience. Some call this "to suck the marrow" out of life. The Explorer wants to find out what it means to live whole-heartedly and fully.

The Explorer seeks to create something out of nothing. Penetrating means to move into spaces that did not exist before in an act of creation. It may be the creating of a family, a business, a team or a safe environment. It may be creating justice where there was injustice. Where there was nothing, your intentional actions made something.

The Explorer will face obstacles as he penetrates the world. Expect significant pushback as you move. This is the normal procedure. Your woman will test you. Nature will test you. Your resolve will be tested. What are you made of? Will you give in? What really brings true meaning and value in your life?

➲ **Penetrate The Void with courage, intent and passion.**

The Initiator Muscle

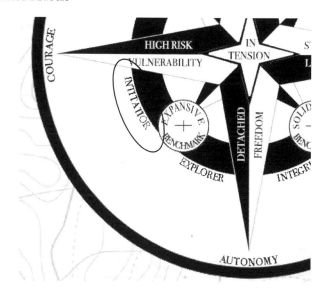

The Initiator Muscle

In the Expansive quadrant and leaning toward the side of Courage and Vulnerability is the Initiator Muscle. The Initiator is very near the top hemisphere that has to do with relationship but is still on the Autonomy side. This means that while the Initiator predominantly has to do with independence and autonomy, he does much of his work in the realm of relationships.

To initiate means to cause something to happen. The Initiator is the agent or cause of actions, experiences or types of environments. He is the cause of action or activity in that he has the courage to choose a certain path of action. He is the cause of experiences in that he is willing to create opportunities for living life to the fullest. He is the agent for creating environments of fun, safety or justice.

We have a very limited amount of power or control in life. Really, we can only control ourselves and only some of what happens in our environment. We can choose to act, not act or how to act. We can choose to make and hold a space for a certain thing like a conversation, loving act or just a secure place to be. The Initiator understands his limitations, but he takes full advantage of the power and control that he does have.

As an influencer, the Initiator can and will take the people around him to new and exciting places of love, experience and play. He is open and vulnerable with his heart to those closest to him.

Courage is the primary characteristic of the Initiator. He is willing to face his fears and move in spite of those fears. He understands that negative things like rejection could be a possibility, but he moves ahead regardless. He will start the difficult conversation, he will ask for help when needed, he will flirt and he will ask for what he needs or wants. He makes things happen.

Here are some other ways the Initiator is defined.

Active/Engaging; The Initiator moves, goes and makes things happen. He just does it and gets it done. He is helpful, emotionally present, affectionate, humorous, and fun. He collaborates and partners with others as a good team-mate and leader. He is appreciative, responsive, interactive, interdependent, reliant, asks for help, and is good at teamwork because he knows it's one of the best ways to get things done. He blesses others, speaks clearly, and listens. The Initiator ascertains what is going on around him, with others he is with and self-ascertains what is going on inside of himself. He is an activator.

Intentional/Purposeful; The Initiator hopes, dreams, is visionary, leads and has develops a plan as he goes through each day. He creates and develops the life he wants and makes it so. He is willing to take the gamble as a lover, an influencer and as an entrepreneur. He develops mastery in many arenas of life. He makes a legacy as he develops his career, builds his family and serves his community. He lives at a balanced pace, is responsible for his actions, creates freedom for himself and others. As life comes to a close, he finishes well.

Life-giving; The Initiator procreates as he begets generativity and creates love, family and blessing. He is observant, aware, and speaks life in as many areas as he can. He is connected, and enlivens relationships through his personal generosity. He is culturally aware and therefore begets freedom, protects innocence, creates environments for growth and innocence as he places self in positions to protect and provide. He creates life out of chaos, bringing order to situations in which he is present. A Greek word, *eudaimonia* fits him well, it means "to create a life of thriving and happiness".

Other Words Describing the Initiator

The Initiator is also a starter, action-oriented, presider, observant, aware, self-confronts, emotionally present, affectionate, reaching, touches, teacher, captain, focused, partners, awake, present, makes you so glad he has chosen you.

The Initiator TLA

MSH = Make Shit Happen

The Initiator makes things happen is his life. He is a starter, he has intent, he follows through and gets stuff done. He is reliable. You can count on him. You want this man on your team. If the zombie apocalypse happened, you would want this guy to be with you. He makes shit happen.

Women love this type of man because they don't have to always make the decisions. They don't have to guess what he wants or needs. They don't have to be responsible. Your woman can rest and enjoy the ride because you are making what needs to happen, happen.

The Expansive Archetype; Creator

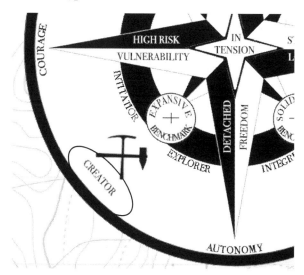

The Creator Archetype

Like any of the archetypes, there are many different things that you think of when you consider the idea of a Creator. A Creator makes something out of nothing. I have spoken of this before, but the most important aspect of the Creator is the concept of "Ex Nihilo". "Ex" is Latin for "out of" just like the English word "exit". "Nihilo" means "nothing", just like "nihilism" which is the belief in nothing or "annihilate" to make something into nothing.

Biblical scholars use this term to describe how God, the Creator, created our world, Ex Nihilo or "out of nothing". The Creator archetype goes back to the beginning of time and makes something out of nothing. Our greatest inventors, writers and imaginative minds have been able to make something out of nothing. Tolkien created Middle Earth with all the history, language, religion, culture and peoples. Da Vinci created the Mona Lisa and many inventions. Benjamin Franklin created many cultural ideas as well as inventions. The Creator is one who takes nothing and makes something.

⮑ **What exists in this world, because you exist?**

Becoming a Creator requires that you know that you have the capacity to create, that you have been designed to make something out of nothing. This is our design, this thing is in us since we have been made in the image of God. Embracing the archetype of Creator is a Godly endeavor.

Becoming a father is becoming a Creator. Your kids did not exist before you did what you needed to do to connect your seed to an egg. This is the same as you create a family. There is now a group of people who live together that never was there before. You can make your family become what you want it to be. Your family of origin may have had characteristics that you did not appreciate, now you have the influence to make your own family become what you want it to be.

The Creator takes up the cause of creating life and then move life toward thriving. His voice is powerful as he actually speaks life into existence by saying what needs to be said, by blessing others, by saying "no", by holding fast to what is right, by standing up. His voice is influential and creates a space of safety and goodness.

Any kind of art or mastery is the realm of the Creator. You can create music, stories, woodwork, houses, buildings, inventions, roads, ideas, photos, paintings, sculpture, events, businesses, new ways to play football (or any sport), new laws, curriculum, apps, software, the list is endless and is only limited by your passion.

Art usually comes from a deep desire to make things more beautiful. Paintings are obvious to this, but engineering a bridge is as well. Or creating a device that will help someone with Type One diabetes to thrive is creating beauty as well. Beauty and thriving are significant goals of the Creator.

Mastery is similar since equipping yourself to become proficient in any endeavor (guitar, electrician, running, coaching, speaking, martial arts, etc.) is how you become a stronger and more influential Creator. What will you choose to master as you become a more powerful Creator?

Being a Force for Good is a man being a Creator. Dr. Jordan B. Peterson challenges us with this question; "Are you tilting the world a little toward hell, or a little toward heaven?" It's a simple question that challenges what kind of man we will be in the universe. A Creator creates and makes something out of nothing. The evil man tilts things toward hell by making something into nothing.

Redemptive Creativity is another type of creating. Redemption is the "buying back" something that was lost. Many of us have estranged relationships where we no longer interact with a family member or friend. This may be for good reasons where you set healthy boundaries. But usually broken relationships are not because of healthy reasons. Redeeming the relationship and healing what is broken is the work of a Creator.

The Creator also creates environments. He holds space to create safety, learning, healing, conversations, play or fun. This can expand to highly influential arenas; creating a concert hall, safety for an entire nation, logistics for making sure food is available, or less grand with having a quiet family meal or a romantic moment with your woman.

Consider the many ways you can begin to expand your ability to create. What do you want to build? How would you want life to be, for you and your family? What do you want to make more beautiful?

Distortions of Quadrant #3

The dark side of Quadrant #3 has three main pitfalls; Passivity, Oblivious and the Domestic. These shadows of Expansiveness, Exploring, Initiating and Creating are so obvious in our world today. Most men don't have many experiences that follow an expansive path. Most men sit back and let much of life just happen. Let's look at these three distortions of a significant part of our manhood, Expansive.

Passivity is described as a life that is frozen, paralyzed, disengaged, inactive, avoidant or withdrawn. This is a living a life which has no Courage to face the vulnerabilities with all the risk that unfolds throughout life. Remember it is not an accident that this quadrant is represented by penetration and metaphorically living with a "hard-on". Therefore, the distortion is as though a man's frame or posture in life is flaccid, limp and unable to move into life with purpose and positive influence.

⤴ **Procrastination is the passive man's limp motivation.**

Often a man will feel "Damned if I do, damned if I don't" and so he just doesn't engage and withdraws. He will get push-back, tension or face obstacles, but since he is dominated by fear of rejection, not getting it right or not being liked, he removes himself from the potential failure by withdrawal or passivity, which becomes a self-fulfilling prophecy and failure to be masculine. As he sits back in his fear, his life passes by and he misses grand opportunities. But it is never too late to change that, by getting into the game.

Oblivious is described as a life that is intentionally or unintentionally being unaware or putting your "head in the sand". The oblivious man is unaware of himself, his own internal workings and his own needs and wants, as well as the wants and needs of those around him. He is ok with the "blue-pill" life and rather uninterested in reality and truth and is content with what he "think"'s is reality and truth.

The oblivious man is satisfied with not being aware, therefore not responsible for action or failure. He does not want ownership or responsibility and since he is off the hook, his woman and others around him become over-responsible. Just like passivity, this is a fear-based posture which keeps a man disengaged, waiting and withdrawn from life.

This means to be aware and conscious, to have your eyes open to the way things really are or to clearly see and understand the experience of others that are different than you. The oblivious man has no need or desire to be awake. He is just fine in his little life, trying to make things work like he always has.

The Domestic is to be tamed or to have your "wildness" driven from your soul. Masculinity has a strong sense of being wild or living freely. The "Wildman" lives deeply within us and is suppressed in our culture, as though there is something wrong or unsafe about him. He was fine in the frontier of the "old west" but not here in town with civilized folk. So, he doesn't have a home, except in a cage.

Most men live in a family context. In the home, the Domestic swallows everything in its path and takes the Wild with it. We get caught up in the logistics, the needs of kids, the honey-do list and keeping things going that we lose a deep part of our soul which is represented by this quadrant. I'm not saying that we don't engage in the Domestic parts of life, that is a huge part of living. Of course, do the dishes, fix the plumbing, change the diapers, take your kid to soccer, but do not, under any circumstances let the Domestic steal your soul.

The Domestic takes hold by taking the easy path, following what you "should" do, making sure everyone is happy with you and having what a perfectly put-together life looks like. That's how it takes over, it gets your attention on what seems to be the most important and then sucks you in. If you will develop the Expansive life you will need to face the Domestic with intent and Courage. The Domestic is a great place to expand your life, you just can't let it take over.

Because most men have never really considered what a life filled with Expansive energy looks like, these three pitfalls or distortions are to be taken seriously. You must consider how to change the entire trajectory of the way you live and then make it happen.

Benchmark #3 Motto:

"I am a man of action, I will move into life intentionally with courage, giving and experiencing as much of life and abundance that I can, in all situations."

Concrete Steps to Build Expansiveness:

Responsibility

> ➔ I am responsible for my life and I will engage in strong personal boundaries.

You are responsible for getting your butt out there, Penetrating the Void and Making Shit Happen. No one else will go in the direction you will go or do this the way you will do it. You will make your own indelible mark on this world, so make it yours. You don't need permission to move and go, just do it like you do it.

Self-Care

⌐ʻ To maintain personal integrity, I must engage in intentional and consistent self-care.

As you engage in Expansiveness your well-being is of prime importance. Remember the guy in the wingsuit shooting through the tiny arch in the video? Yeah, he will probably die young. The saying goes, there are bold climbers and there are old climbers, but there are no old bold climbers. So, as you get out there and explore and initiate and create, be wise and choose well. Prepare yourself well for whatever endeavor you seek. As always get in shape, get the sleep you need and eat well.

Balance

⌐ʻ Keeping a good balance in life will help me hold my center.

If you choose to be a husband or a father, keep strong balance with your adventures and your providing/protecting. If you remain single or kidless, just remember you do have people who love you, so respect their desire to keep you safe. Give them regard, but don't let that keep you from moving and expanding.

Now we will move from expanding your world and your outer experience to creating a life of Passion as we develop our final quadrant.

Questions; Quadrant Three is at the crossroads of Autonomy and Courage, where we become a man of action, moving into life intentionally with courage, giving <u>and</u> experiencing as much of life and abundance that I can, in all situations. This Quadrant has the Muscles of Explorer and Initiator, the TLA's of Penetrate The Void (PTV) and Make Shit Happen (MSH) and the Archetype of Creator.

What seems like the most important aspect for you to build?

Balancing the realities of High Risk, Vulnerability and Courage with Autonomy and being the best version of yourself, means that you will place your self out into the dangerous world. Whether that is through adventure, relationship, business, or just playing with life, it will be getting out there and creating the life you want. In what ways have you been doing this, or not?

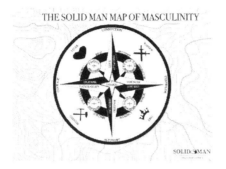

THE SOLID MAN MAP OF MASCULINITY

8 Quadrant Four - Passion

We are now on our last quadrant. From the individual or autonomy hemisphere, we are moving up into the relational hemisphere, so this quadrant brings us back into our interactions with others. We remain in the High-Risk side of life where Vulnerability, danger and discomfort exist. This is the corner where Courage meets Connection.

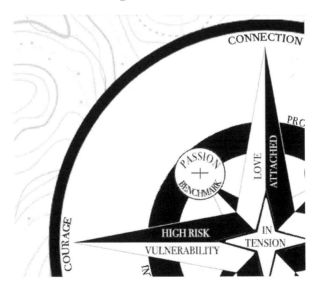

The Passion Benchmark

The word that represents this quadrant is Passion.

The concept of Passion is deeper than what it seems, so it takes some explanation. When you hear the word Passion, you probably think of love, desire, romance, lust or sexuality. These are absolutely concepts of Passion, however there is so much more.

Like so many concepts, think of Passion as a coin with two sides. The first side is desire and the second side is emptiness or suffering.

The desire side of Passion is ruled by the instinctive parts of our system; heart, intuitive, emotional, gut. As we move through life, we accumulate things we desire that are not from choice or necessarily from our conscious awareness. For instance, we may be attracted to blondes or brunettes, not out of choice, but just because. This is true of all the millions of other things we may desire; breasts v. butts, Ford v. Chevy, peace v. adrenaline, etc. At times desire comes from unexplainable places.

Passion is desire, and desire at its core is wanting. Desire as a concept requires not having something. If you had that thing you would no longer desire or long for it because it is now in your possession. So, Passion as desire is wanting or longing for some thing.

Since I want something, I don't have that thing and so as my want and desire increase, it becomes Passion; where my energy, focus and intent are increasing toward that which I don't have (desire). The big question here is "What do you want?" So many people go through life more concerned with what everybody else wants, or what will make them happy – with me. To ask, "What do I want?" is selfish, therefore it is not ok to desire. This is wrong.

The masculine man knows what he wants and pursues that. You may not achieve what you desire, that's not the point. The point is allowing yourself to live with desire, with the wanting. Remember just because you desire something does not mean it needs to be or will be fulfilled. Living with desire is where Passion comes alive. Passion is defined by desire or wanting, not necessarily the fulfillment of that desire.

Which brings us to the other side of the coin, Passion is emptiness or embracing sacrifice or embracing not having something. We usually do everything we can to fill or fulfill all of our desires without even thinking about it. The emptiness aspects of Passion require that we are attentive to our desire and aware of our experience of wanting. We are required to allow our conscious to enter the game and become attentive and aware of what we actually desire. Our maturity and self-discipline in the realm of Passion is borne from emptiness.

Emptiness is having serenity and peace in a state of not having something, yet not having to fill any emptiness or void. Embracing emptiness is intentional self-sacrifice from a place of strength for the good of others [love]. Passion requires that you embrace the fears and anxieties of life, not escape from them or numb them out. So often when men experience emptiness or tension, they will turn to their drug of choice to feel better. This is an escape from feeling empty and not experiencing the fullness of Passion, you'll never feel much Passion about life at all.

➔ We will often turn to any "Drug of Choice" to escape emptiness.

Purposefully pursuing the emptiness of Passion is a brilliant movement which truly clarifies the desires of a man. You may have been pursuing what you want, which is good. Now as emptiness is experienced a man is able to consciously decide "Is this what I **really** want?" This is about clarity. Embracing the tension that emptiness brings helps you to determine what is of true value to you in your life, what you spend your limited energy and Passion on attaining what has real meaning to you.

The challenge to embrace emptiness and desire at the same time, will allow you to experience the fulness of deep living. Your life will become more alive, purposeful and full. The emotions you stuffed, the empathy you set aside and the love you want will come back deeply. To some this is a daunting excursion and takes Courage, that's Passion.

So, on one hand Passion creates a posture of excitement and drive where a man energetically pursues that which he desires. And on the other hand, he is able to rest in the tension of not having that which he desires (emptiness). He does not have to possess or own anything to experience wholeness and contentment in life.

Healthy Passion is experienced in a beautiful balance between drive and desire with suffering and emptiness. Unhealthy Passion is a compulsive drive to possess, which is addiction. Unhealthy Passion will have nothing to do with emptiness, it must possess whatever it is that it desires. Healthy Passion can rest in the desire of not having.

➔ Passion = the balance of desire and emptiness.

This is difficult for men who have turned away from desire. It may be that you have been taught that desire is sinful, or at least some of the things you desire are sinful, like the shape of a woman's body or the sexual energy that is described as feeling horny.

So, you have spent much of your life pushing desires down and seeing yourself as defective. So many men question their God-given sex drive.

You may have been rejected or abandoned, so desiring to be in a close relationship puts you in a position that feels very dangerous, as if life really is at stake. Your desire for intimacy forces you to move into the emptiest place of your life. Because it feels dangerous you will then just hold back.

Living with Passion is no small endeavor. Consider one of the most significant stories which uses the word Passion; The Passion of the Christ. Most people are puzzled by the fact that the term "Passion" is used for this story. For us, men who are wanting to live to the fulness of Masculinity, it makes sense. It is the perfect example of what it would mean to experience Passion in every sense of the word.

Christ was at once moving with the deep desire and love for humanity while experiencing one of the most grueling deaths mankind has devised. The desire for the well-being and relationship for people is driving his willingness to allow himself to be crucified. It is Passion, as both desire and emptiness are at play simultaneously.

This sacrifice as Passion is a willingness to place yourself in suffering or harm's way for others. This is not a self-harm or suicidal mentality, but an attitude of fearless courage for the well-being of those you love. A man could only do this if he has somewhat settled the specter of death that floats around our lives. This man can choose to give his life as sacrifice, whether that is losing his life in full by taking a bullet or choosing to use his time to help his kid with homework rather than watching the ball game.

This is where the two Cornerstones are interacting as well. The desire for Connection is the driver and the movement is one of Courage and Vulnerability. Christ spends his greatest Commodity for the souls of all humans. In this extremely vulnerable action he commits by dying on the cross, was one of the most powerful acts in human history. This is Passion.

Whereas the story of Jesus is powerful and even extreme, how would any regular man live a life of Passion? What would this look like? Using the language of the Map of Masculinity, a man of Passion would live with Courage as he seeks Connection. The man of Passion would fearlessly be whole-hearted, open and engaged in all he does; relationships, adventure, play, work, and calling. He pursues what he desires, but is ok if he does not obtain it.

The man of Passion would seek connection, intimacy and restoration of relationships. True, he is limited with only having so much bandwidth in relationships, but those he has committed to, he does in full.

Other Words that Describe Passionate: embraces emptiness, gives, loves, cares, makes personal sacrifices, listens, sees, cherishes, speaks, blesses, pays attention to self and others, vulnerable, open, empathetic, compassionate, attentive, knows his emotions and feelings, redemptive, patient, committed, faithful, supports, gracious, graceful, thankful, content, reliable, pursues and is settled.

The two Muscles of the Passion Quadrant will give more meat to the idea of what it means to live with Passion, so let's take a look at those Muscles; Thumos and Eros.

The Thumos Muscle

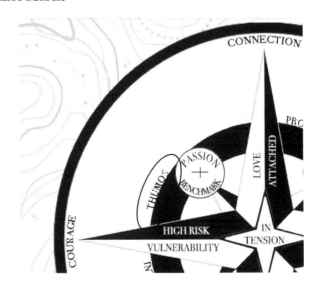

The Thumos Muscle

In the Passion quadrant and leaning toward the cornerstone of Courage and Vulnerability is the Thumos Muscle. Thumos is in the top hemisphere that has to do with Relationship but leans toward the Courage Cornerstone. This means that while Thumos predominantly has to do with a man of Courage and Vulnerability, he does much of his work in the realm of connection and relationships.

The ancient Greek philosophers spoke of Thumos as a life-force found in certain things, like a spirited stallion or a spirited debate. Here, I am using the word Thumos to define that aspect of a man that is spirited, vigorous and full of vitality. It is having a strong sense of enthusiasm about life.

Thumos describes a man who lives with a whole heart being present and aware and open with all he does. Since this part of the quadrant leans toward Courage, it is more to do with a man's posture in life, that he is open and courageous as he moves into life.

Philosopher Allan Bloom called Thumos "the central natural passion in men's souls." As a driving and energizing force, Thumos is a powerful aspect of a man's presence in his own life. Consider men from history or from your own life who have this strong presence. They seem to be a little bigger than life and you know they are in the room.

Remember the quote in *The Abolition of Man*, C.S. Lewis said, "In a sort of ghastly simplicity we remove the organ and demand the function. We make men without chests and expect of them virtue and enterprise. We laugh at honour and are shocked to find traitors in our midst. We castrate and bid the geldings be fruitful."

Men with "chests" have Thumos. Men with virtue and enterprise have Thumos. Unfortunately, something that our culture has achieved, rather successfully, is to have created men who are void of Thumos. Removing Thumos is the equivalent of castration, yet the double standard exists that the culture still would say, "Man up!" while not having Thumos.

It is only through revitalizing the presence of Thumos will we ever be able to really live as men, as we have been designed. The "organ" that has been removed is our heart, our vitality, our Thumos. Even though we have been cut off from this important part of our Masculinity, it can be reclaimed. We must begin to exercise the Muscle of Thumos.

Brett McKay from The Art of Manliness says it this way, "Yet in our modern day, instead of helping men to harness their thumos for positive ends, society has decided it is better to neuter the force altogether. To protect some people from getting hurt, we've tried to breed it out of men, even if it means its positive effects will be sacrificed along with the negative. It is like getting rid of electricity, and all the benefits that have come with it, because some people get electrocuted."

Thumos comes alive when you are aroused, moved, and emotional. Thumos is when you are responsive to beauty, truth, goodness and justice.

It is righteous indignation and it is a sweet, gentle touch. It is excitement at the start of an adventure and it is eye contact during a job interview. It is being moved to tears at a good friend's funeral and it is the awe you experience when you see a beautiful sunset or a beautiful ballet.

Thumos is the driver that makes us get up to do something and stand up for something. It is a motivator and an instigator. It is a deep internal aliveness that pushes us toward adventure, love and engagement. It is the drive into purpose and discovering why the hell you are on this planet. You will find your purpose if you live with Thumos. Thumos will come alive in your soul and your Passion and purpose will become clear.

A man with Thumos will create an environment of safety but also tension. He will "hold space" with whatever energy is in the room. He is able to be present and remain present in whatever situation he is in. People know him as engaging since he will interact with intent with those around him. Sure, he may be an introvert, but he is engaged with life and people.

When it is called for, he will stand firm and rise up. He is ready and prepared because he is aware of what is going on. He holds fast to all he sees as dear to him and is willing to speak up when necessary.

The Muscle of Thumos is as necessary as the rest of the Muscles, but some men have a tough time exercising this one. Just like the Cornerstones of the quadrant suggest it requires Courage and Connection. Thumos is totally connected with life and it takes tons of Courage to live with that kind of Passion.

Words that describe Thumos are;

Vitality; Vitality is a word that says a man is full of life. He has liveliness and is highly spirited. He is described as energetic and alive. He is engaged and interactive with people and with experience. He just enjoys life and is very present.

A man with vitality is expressive with his words and actions, not being overly verbose or talkative, but also listening and being curious. He is not so concerned with his own business, but he is engaged with the world where he wants to experience it all. This is the classic "sucking the marrow" out of life motif. He is very alive.

Driven; A man with Thumos has an internal drive and motivation. He gets things done. His drive comes from the depth of his purpose and desires. He knows what he wants, and moves to make that happen. It could be work or it could be relationship, regardless of the context, he is active to make it so.

Temperance/Discipline; As Passion has two sides, so does Thumos. As much as a man is full of drive, he is also aware of not having or sacrifice. He is able to withhold, wait or go without. This is temperance, choosing to not have something, when you want it. At times a man of Thumos will live in simplicity or without many things. He will choose to be stoic in nature. He will seek the building of his endurance with discipline and work. He does this with choice and Passion.

Fearless/Settled; This seems very paradoxical, but he lives life in a "Today is a good day to die" way. The big questions of life are fairly settled. No man can know fully what will come when we die, but a man with Thumos embraces death with dignity. He has settled that he will die and made provisions for that as he has seen fit, which allows for Thumos.

Having settled the ultimate question, he can now live fully with fearlessness or Courage in all he does. This is a huge part of Thumos. He can pursue all he wants to with fullness and depth, with Vulnerability and openness, with all of his heart.

Other Words that Describe Thumos;

Thumos is also sturdiness, toughness, hardiness, strength, spiritedness, internal urge, conscious, aware, creates, builds, motivated, ownership, responsible, vision, reliable, count-on-able, , honor and purpose, self-discipline, endurance, intentional, purposeful, not filling the void, purposeful, aware of the sacred, unfinished, unknowing, embrace mystery, doesn't have to control, lives in tension, anchored, influential, fully alive.

The Thumos TLA

LWH = Live Whole Hearted

The man with Thumos lives with a whole heart. This means his heart is open to all that life has, profound and difficult. He embraces life and love, as well as discipline and grief. He is as integrated with as much of his internal resources as possible, open and aware of his deep internal workings. He is as connected to experiences, community and family to the fullest degree he is capable.

Whole Hearted living is the mark of a man with Thumos. He is connected to life and lives life to the fullest by opening his heart to what life brings. He seeks thriving and abundance for himself and all who join with him.

The Eros Muscle

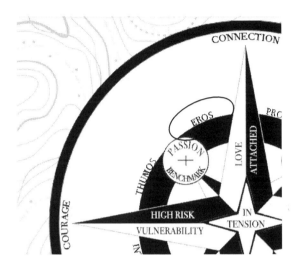

The Muscle of Eros

In the Passion quadrant and leaning toward the cornerstone of Connection and Love is the Eros Muscle. Eros is in the top hemisphere that has to do with Relationship and is involved with the aspects of life that are about Love, Connection and Attachment. This means that while Eros predominantly has to do with the realm of Connection and Relationships he still is involved with Courage and Vulnerability.

Eros is a Greek word that is one of the four Greek words found in the Bible that define Love. *Storge* is the family bond type of Love. *Phileo* is a friendship connection as in *"philadelphia"* or "brotherly love", *phileo* is love and *delphos* is brother. *Agape* is the type of Love that is unconditional, sacrificial and pure.

Eros represents the sexual, sensual, romantic, passionate Love of desire and physical attraction. I am using it here in the Passion Quadrant as the word describing the masculine Muscle which is very connected in relationship and very open with Courage and Vulnerability. A man who lives strong with the Muscle of Eros is living a life that is Passionate (desire and sacrifice), open and connected. It is about sexual arousal and so much more.

> ➔ **Eros is life energy that comes out of us to create life.**

Whereas the Thumos muscle is in a man's passion for life and living full, Eros is a man's passion for connection, intimacy and relationship. A significant aspect of being human is the fact that life is the inescapable context of relationships. We cannot escape this. For a human, relationships are similar to the air we breathe in that it we are bathed in it every moment, we need it to keep living well and often we are oblivious to our interactions with it.

Since we are engaged in relationships on a daily, even hourly basis, if we are going to live well and with intention, we must become aware of our interactions, our own necessity for relationships and the ways in which we do relationships in healthy and unhealthy ways. Considering the Muscle of Eros will help to make things clear.

As the word Eros is usually used for our sexuality and romantic interactions, I am using about general relationships as well. It would be the drive for building a strong family, it is about building your Mt. Rushmore with the men you want to have in your life, it is building any relationship that has deeper and stronger bonds than the normal interactions you have on a daily basis.

Your relationships with your children and members of your family of origin are the close relationships that you will pursue and develop as you embrace the Muscle of Eros. The Passion a man has for his children is a beautiful example of this muscle at play. Be passionate and engaged with your kids, it is one of the most beautiful expressions of our Masculinity.

Jack Donovan speaks of building your tribe or gang of men. Men who will be with you in thick and thin. Men that have proven themselves as those who will have your back when things get bad. This is your Band of Brothers, men who are with you in life. This has nothing to do with romance or sex, but it has everything to do with passion and brotherhood. It is a deep sense of love. It is the *"phileo"* love, but I am also speaking that there is a more passionate aspect to it as well. Every man must build his tribe.

This may seem odd, but this is where you would develop closeness in an intimate relationship with God, or your Source, however you see things. Many men desire to develop a deep relationship with their creator and this relationship intimacy is expressed in the realm of Eros. It is deeply intimate and passionate, not as lovers or in any form of sexuality, but it is close, intimate and anchored.

But mostly, the Muscle of Eros is reserved for your relationship with your woman. She is the one who will receive your focus, desire and commitment like no other. This is not putting her on a pedestal as a goddess but reserving your energy and passion for her above other women. There is something deeply sacred within a marriage, so pursuing and penetrating your woman's heart, soul and body is divine.

Eros allows you to be known, to be seen for who you really are. You are able to know and to see the other as well. This deep soul-level intimacy is the essence of Eros.

⊙ **Love is the PRIME virtue.**

Remember the main idea of the word Eros is about love. Love has always been the highest virtue in our world. Love is the Prime virtue. Of all the virtues I have been presenting, love, either Thumos and the zest for life or Eros and the passion for connection and relationship, brings depth and fulness into our lives like nothing else.

⊙ **Love brings life like nothing else.**

What I am saying is that a strong, driven, passionate, and engaged Masculinity is what the Muscle of Eros is all about. Here are some words that describe Eros more fully.

Vigor; A man who expresses Eros is alive. His movements, intentions and behaviors are full of energy and vitality. There is a fervor in his steps and choices. This may sound like he moves impulsively, it is not, he moves with life and passion. Not sure how else to say it, his life is full of life. That's what vigor is.

Engaged; The man of Eros is engaged. He has entered into relationships with a connectedness and openness. He is aware of the deep value of connectedness and therefore moves into relationships with intent and clarity. Even though they are often a space of the sacred, relationships become a place of play as well. He is able to remain in rest in the deep moments of gravity and also teasing in lighter moments of laughter and ease. He is engaged.

Sexual; Eros is a very sexy aspect of living. Engaging in Eros fully means that a man has processed his shame around his sexuality. Many of us have a sense that sexuality is dirty or wrong, that our drive or desire for sex reveals something is deeply broken or wrong within you. To become a man who is free, you must overcome this bondage.

A man's sexuality is one of his most profound arenas of influence as well as his enjoyment of life. Sex covers the full display of human living from physical pleasure to emotional connection to transcendent worship. It is a beautiful thing that adds so much to the gift of life.

Desire; Having a strong feeling of wanting something or for something to happen is desire. Wanting is desire. Many men have either forgotten their desires, lost permission to want or have pushed aside their desires as if their desires are bad. Desire might be seen as selfish or sinful, therefore must be disregarded. This is a huge pitfall, if you lose your desire you lose your ability to want. When you lose your wants, you lose the ability to choose or lead your own life in freedom.

Desire and Eros are so intertwined. Eros is wanting something, whether that is sex or connection or fulfilling purpose. The roots of desire are deep within one's heart and soul. It is true that sometimes we might want something in an impulsive or foolish way, but that says more about how we choose rather than what we desire or what we most desire. For instance, I may desire to have sex with random women, but my greater desire is to have a strong marriage, so I choose my path with one woman.

- **Desire is good, wanting is good.**

Pursuit; Going after the things we desire is significant as well. Sitting passively is not how Masculinity is lived out. Passivity and procrastination are the opposite of pursuit. Pursuing what you want and either making it happen or reaching out and getting it, is masculine.

Most women want to be pursued. It means that you care, that you think she is attractive, that you are aroused by her, that she is beautiful, that she impacts your life. She wants to know she rocks your world. She will test you and push back, that's part of the pursuit, she wants to know that you have resolve and will keep up the pursuit. It is play, it is flirting, it is tension. Pursuit is Eros in action.

Sacrifice; The other side of the coin of Passion was the pain that comes from loving and being connected. The more connection and love you feel, the more pain you may experience. Let's say you become very attached to your woman after years of open conversation, deep and meaningful love-making, building a family and pursuing dreams. You are attached. But as life has it, someone will die.

- **The more you open yourself up to love, the more pain you will feel.**

Since someone will die, either you or her, someone will feel the most intense loss imaginable. Not only will you make sacrifices to work hard or go without things periodically, you will experience grief. I think I am saying the same thing as Buddhism that attachment is suffering. However, with a different angle, I am saying living with Eros means that you will choose to attach deeply and therefore choose to suffer deeply. Eros, like Passion, is suffering as well, however it is suffering with deep meaning and intent.

Other words that Describe Eros;

Eros can also be seen as lover, aroused, desire, connecting, attentive, seductive, flirty, robustness, health, horniness, intensity, focus, potent, gusto, hard-on, hardiness, stamina, play, fun, energizing, laughter, caring, heart, restlessness, alive, openness, empathetic, passionate, compassionate, attentive, knows and values emotions and feelings, liveliness, energetic, survivor, aware of and healed from wounds, longing, pursuit, appetite, motivated, generous, wants, undone, serenity in want, surrender, suffering, vulnerability, cherishing, delighting, blessing, open, embracing not having and being ok with it because there is a true Source of life, embraces purposeful emptiness , committed, and faithful.

The Eros TLA

PIP= Pursue Intimacy Passionately

The man with Eros pursues intimacy with Passion. He goes after (pursues) closeness and connection (intimacy) with intention and courage (passionately). Eros is a driver of deep meaningful connection.

Intimacy is a state of openness to allow someone to see you. I've heard this way of describing intimacy; "In-To-Me-See". I know it is cheesy, but it describes letting someone in to your inner world, they now have seen and have your heart. You have chosen to spend your Vulnerability currency in this way with this person.

⤳ Love is the Prime Virtue and Intimacy is the doorway.

The man of Eros recognizes the deep life meaning of intimacy and then goes after it with vigor and vulnerability which takes a strong measure of courage. You trust the ones you choose to be open with and give them permission to know the true you.

Pursue Intimacy Passionately (PIP) is a call to live life with deep Eros Love. It is open and vulnerable. It is alive and free. It is connected and togetherness. It is one of the most terrifying and yet one of the most beautiful experiences of life.

The Archetype of Quadrant Four; Lover

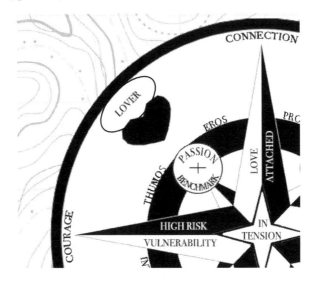

Passion Quadrant Archetype; The Lover

The Lover Archetype

There are many people in literature and history that hold the Lover archetype. People like Romeo and Juliet, Sir Lancelot and Guinevere, Romeo and Juliet, Rhett Butler and Scarlett O'Hara, Elizabeth Bennett and Mr. Darcy and Rose and Jack from Titanic. There are the classic lovers Valentino, Don Juan, the Phantom of the Opera or Casanova. Or one's you don't often consider as the Lover archetype like Dracula or Pepe le Pew.

The Lover is a very common and important aspect of most literature. There usually is some sort of love going on. If not, it's kind of boring. The funky pseudo incest between Luke and Leia Skywalker made things interesting until Han Solo stole Leia's heart. Even The Lord of the Rings had Samwise Gamgee and Rosie Cotton and Aragorn and Arwen as side stories to keep it interesting. The Lover is everywhere, especially thriving in bad literature.

The Lover seeks connection and intimacy. Building relationships is a significant pastime. These relationships could be romantic, but they are also platonic or networking types of relationships with no intent to be sexual. It is about being with others. It could be in the context of sexual and romantic, it could be business and entrepreneurial, it could be sports and competition or it could be in a gang or a tribe.

⮞ **The Lover seeks and thrives in being with others.**

The Lover is sensuous, in that he is awake to all his physical, emotional, spiritual and relational processes. He notices what is happening and holds space in as many experiences as possible. The Lover has an enthusiastic appetite for living, for passion and experiences of all types. This is the Thumos side of the Lover, moving into life with excitement and intention.

⮞ **The Lover loves living and all that life provides.**

The Lover lives with an open heart because he knows that this is how he will experience life in the fullest. He wants that whole-hearted gusto that exists with openness to all experiences, whether they are fulfilling, joyful or even in grief.

Because of this, the Lover can fall into what looks and feels like depression, they are feeling the rough parts of life fully. Things will potentially become a crisis and as he feels deeply, he will process the experience deeply. This is necessary so that the realities of life will be seen, known and implanted in his soul.

But he also has the capability of feeling the most beautiful and profoundly uplifting parts as well. This will feel like a roller-coaster at times because this is the way life is and the Lover lives life openly.

The Lover often is a seducer and a flirt, being very playful and fun in the arena of relational interaction and comfortable with sexual tension. This is not necessarily to experience sex, but often is, but also just because he enjoys the banter and tension of relational energy.

As a seducer, the Lover seeks and appreciates beauty. The intimacy of a connection with another is profoundly beautiful. He allows himself to rest in awe of anything beautiful; the feminine form, a well-timed joke, a nice move in sports, art that moves him, a sunset, or his child giggling uncontrollably. His attachment to beauty and connection, to intimacy and experience is what defines how he lives life. He is highly attached to all these experiences. They bring depth and fullness to life.

The seducer aspect often is met with disdain because of how many men have used it just to get laid or to take advantage of people. This is true, many have abused this aspect of the Lover. However, when it is engaged with the "Solid Frame" quadrant the seducer is a very healthy aspect of the Masculine. The seducer is one who invites another into the life of thriving, intimacy and enjoying experience. He invites others into life.

> ⟿ **The Lover seduces, and seducing or inviting others into life at its fullest!**

The Lover is not just super out-going as an extrovert but can also be found in the introverted side of personality. As an introvert, the Lover's sense of connection seems to flow much deeper and pursuing a more profound sense of intimacy. He may pour much of his energy into building one deeper relationship rather than into many relationships.

God is often seen as the Lover as he pursues mankind into relationship. Many aspects of Christianity speak to God's Passion for paving a way for intimate relationship with the people he has created. Again this is where the Passion of the Christ is an expression of the love God has for us.

The Lover is the most fragile archetype in Masculinity. As he feels deeply and experiences life openly, he is vulnerable to pain and loss. That's what Vulnerability is. He is putting himself "out there" in life so he has a high potential for negative experience. This is where seeking the wisdom of spending currencies of Love and Vulnerability is essential.

The Lover must connect deeply to his Solid Frame (King) archetype to maintain groundedness. The balance of all the masculine quadrants is necessary to master Masculinity, this creates an "anti-fragile" life.

Passion Quadrant Motto:

"I will live with an Open Heart, pursuing life and love with energy, intent, purpose and fearless passion and at times sacrifice, when I don't receive what I desire, I will embrace the emptiness of "not having" with grace and maturity."

Distortions of Quadrant #4 Passion –

The dark side of Quadrant #4 has three main pitfalls; **Closed Heart, Impulsivity/Compulsivity** and **Abuse**. These shadows of Passion, Thumos, Eros and the Lover are not that obvious as distortions because they are more normal or expected of men than not. Most men dramatically fall into these distortions without even thinking about what they are doing.

Let's look at these three distortions of Passionate manhood.

A Closed Heart is the opposite of having an open heart. An open heart is open to experience and love, but also potential pain and suffering. A closed heart is lead by fearfulness and self-protection. It is generally seen in a defensive or victim posture. The closed heart therefore disengages and withdraws from life, from relationship and from any experience that may be difficult or uncomfortable. This results in a life that is unconscious, blank, powerless and generally dead to abundance.

A closed heart also has alexithymia. Remember, alexithymia is that fancy word for not being in touch with your emotions. When you close off to any outside pain, you also close off to any of your vital internal resources as well. This closes you off to yourself as well as others. Whatever you've been taught about emotions, it is very, very unwise to close them off. You must engage with your internal resources, your emotional process being one of the most important. Keep an open heart as much as you can in life.

Rather than being ok with closing yourself off, stay emotionally engaged. Men who are emotionally engaged may still look stoic, but they are quite aware of their own emotional processes and vulnerably open with their own emotions with people who are close to them and emotionally safe. They learn that anger is not the thing that controls their lives but is only indicating their well-being; an indicator guiding them to what they need. They have Passion, living with vigor and vitality proceeding from freedom. Passion requires that you embrace the fears and anxieties of life, not escaping from them or numbing them out. It is living a whole-hearted life.

<u>Impulsivity/Compulsivity</u>; This is where a man has limited self-discipline with what he thinks and unconsciously, ritualistically acts to get what he thinks he desires. He will move with impulsivity, acting without thought or intention. He will do things foolishly. Impulsivity is Passion with no internal restraint. It is moving without healthy boundaries, integrity or honor.

Compulsivity is moving and acting according to whatever urges one may have at any given moment. Similar to impulsivity, compulsivity is more about urges that exist from addictions or counterfeits, things that we pursue because we think they will give us life or fill a void within. The man of Passion understands these urges, where they come from and is able to choose emptiness or not having something, with wisdom and self-discipline.

➔ Pursuit of unhealthy desire can easily become addiction.

Impulsive and compulsive behavior is addiction and addiction is desire gone awry. It is our deep desires being played out without wisdom, integrity or the ability to be empty or going without something. Addiction wants to fill the Void with consumerism, possessing something, controlling, using others or substances in addictive absorption to relieve pain or emptiness, with fearful and anxious self-protection. The man of Passion is able to choose to live on the sacrifice and empty side of the Passion coin.

Abuse; Abuse is controlling others and your surroundings in order to achieve a sensation of power. This is played out as "power-over". It is a drive to absorb and to possess things in order to fulfill personal deficit or to compensate for inadequacies.

Although the majority of men reduce their positive influence on the world by refraining from entering into life (passivity), some men will engage in behaviors which abuses those around him. Abuse is improper and unhealthy treatment of a person, where the other person is a tool to for the abuser to achieve a sense of strength that is missing from his internal self. This distortion exists in this quadrant because this is how men without integrity or internal fortitude often relate.

Abuse comes in many forms; physical, sexual, emotional, verbal etc. A man who abuses has chosen to fight against the very people he has been designed to protect. He is fighting a battle against his own Masculinity, hurting those around him rather than providing safety for them. The abuser moves out of self-protectiveness and fear. He uses the strength he has to put those around him into harm, to break them down, with accusation, and exposes them to potential harm. This is POWER OVER but is different in that it is purposefully controlling others, which is a perversion of all the quadrants; Power For, Solid Frame, Expansiveness and Passion.

Concrete Steps to Build Passion:

Responsibility

> ☞ I am responsible for my life and I will engage in strong personal boundaries.

Responsibility is huge in the Passion quadrant. You must be diligent to keep your values and move from your solid core with your values and character leading how you move. Many men have been lost in a maelstrom of wretched relationships because they chose unwisely which women to interact with. Be the one who chooses and chooses well who you might engage with in Passion.

Hold strong with your personal boundaries and don't spend your precious currencies on someone just because they are hot or into you.

Self-Care

➔ To maintain personal integrity, I must engage in intentional and consistent self-care.

Self-care always is important. In relationship and romance, many men give up themselves to keep her happy, or more precisely to keep her happy with him. You can't do this, you must keep your own self-care at the top of your priorities. If she doesn't allow this, then she cannot be the one for you. Passion is about love, romance and connection; you must not lose yourself in that. Keep your frame and your priorities.

Balance

➔ Keeping a good balance in life will help me hold my center.

Like responsibility and self-care, it seems redundant to talk about balance. But as you engage in Passion, if you do not hold fast to your Solid Frame you will lose both your Power and your ability to Expand. So many men lose their soul in this quadrant. There is much to be experienced with Passion, but it must be done while holding fast to your center, your Solid Frame.

Questions; Quadrant Four is at the crossroads of Connection and Courage, living with an Open Heart and pursuing desire with energy, intent and purpose and embracing emptiness. The Muscles of Thumos and Eros, the TLA's of Live Whole Hearted (LWH) and Pursue Intimacy Passionately (PIP) and is represented by the Archetype of the Lover. What seems like the most important aspect for you to build?

Walking the balance between our Connection with the people around us and the Courage to engage with life to the fullest, both in adventure and relationship is a significant part of living out our Masculinity. In what ways has balancing this been difficult or something you're good at?

9 Mastering Masculinity

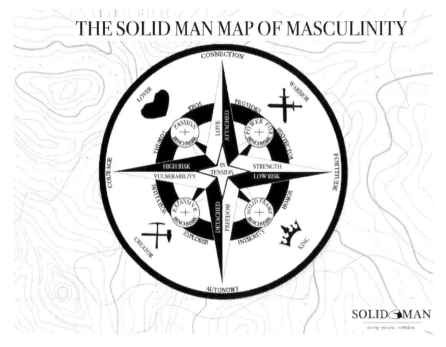

The Solid Man Map of Masculinity

There it is in all its glory, the Solid Man Map of Masculinity with all the working parts. Now your goal is to master it. You've read the concepts, you have seen how each move with the others, and you have a good idea how it plays out in real life. Now the challenge is for you to begin to build proficiency, competence and mastery with this vital internal resource.

Remember that the map is not the territory, you are the territory. You are the land upon which these concepts become real. We all have our own unique topography, so make it your own. With this map, I am giving the skeleton to the structure of how Masculinity will take shape in your life. It's not just giving it the muscles and guts, but you'll give it it's Passion and Vision. Now, let's get to mastering your Masculinity.

Mastery

Mastery is skill, competence or knowledge over a subject or any area of expertise. Many people say that it takes 10,000 hours of deliberate practice, until we begin to master anything. Some say 25,000 hours is more like it.

We are not like the movie *The Matrix*, where things are downloaded into your head, "I know Kung Fu?" It will take time and effort. It is a journey, as well as the destination. (but a destination with which you probably will not be satisfied with in the end, you'll probably still strive for more).

Mastering will require drive, discipline, focus, desire, time, and passion. And for some, depending on the area of mastery, it will seem to come naturally. So then this begs the question; "do you have to be born this way?". Is it the thought that if you got it, you got it or can it be developed? That answer is yes, and yes. But there are limitations.

You do have to have the raw materials. Master basketball like Michael Jordan? Maybe not, since I don't have the body, the drive or the hops. I can enjoy basketball (I actually played very small college ball), but I will never achieve his level of mastery.

⮑ **You will need specific raw materials to master certain things.**

It's the same when I learned the basics of the guitar, but since I do not have much of a sense of rhythm, I could never master that. Which also hindered my ability to master any dancing. My wife and I have enjoyed learning dancing (except for the public humiliation at times), but I could not easily figure out if it was 4/4 or 3/4 time, which determines which kind of dancing you'll choose. So, I'll enjoy it, but never master it.

All that to say is you need the raw materials. We all cheered when Rudy Ruettiger played in the game in *Rudy*, but that was as far as he got with football. I guess he later somewhat mastered a motivational speaking career, good for him. The point is that we do need the tools for that particular arena we wish to master. Some things need a certain level of brain power, some a level of athleticism, some need money, strength, or maybe an intense or laid-back personality. Whatever it is we want to pursue, we must be honest if we have or don't have the raw materials to be able to master that thing.

⮑ **Do not think that what is hard for you to master is humanly impossible; and if it is humanly possible, consider it to be within your reach.   – Marcus Aurelius**

Aurelius is saying that if it is humanly possible, it is in your reach. As a man you have the raw materials to master Masculinity, therefore, it is possible. You may have limitations in some areas, but you have strengths in others. This is how it will become yours. You give it the shape that your own personal interests, strengths, passions, weaknesses, wounds, victories, physical boundaries, gifts, and incompetencies will come together to create.

According to Robert Greene in his book *Mastery*, your path to mastery contains three distinct phases. The first is the Apprenticeship, the second is the Creative-Active, and the third is Mastery itself.

Apprenticeship is the instruction stage. You will do what you can to learn everything you can about that field of study. Here, it is important to find a mentor, a coach or a sage who has been down this road. This stage is the silent, unseen preparation. Learning the basic elements and rules. Going over the fundamentals over and over, again and again; making mistakes, over and over, again and again. This is where you must have the "Beginner's Mind" and just be humble.

This practice stage is often called "Surrender" because you are giving your time and often don't see results. It is Mr. Miyagi telling you to "wax on, wax off", you might lose your motivation because it is tedious, and you don't see the point. You must have willingness to feel awkward, look silly or be incompetent. You must be ok with growing and getting better. You know how incompetent you are, and it helps you move ahead. It will seem rigorous, and it will take dedication and grit.

In the Creative-Active stage you will start to see how things connect with one another. It will feel more like intention. You will slow it down, ingraining it into your muscle memory. Whatever it is, will become a part of you. Brain pathways will begin to shift. Your vision for mastery will become clearer and clearer.

But, in this stage you will plateau. There will be negative feedback loops which want to keep you the same. Something in you will want to keep the old homeostasis, keeping it at 98.6 degrees. You must fight through this and embrace the positive feedback loop which wants the change, wants the new you.

Passion is one thing that will push you through the negative feedback loops. You can't do this without a whole heart or do it half-fast, you have to be all in during this stage or you'll never experience mastery.

You will be pushing the envelope, finding new paths, experiencing new proficiencies, expanding your practice. You see your progress, that you're getting the hang of it, and maybe even feeling competent. Remember you're still in the 10,000 to 25,000 stage.

Then comes Mastery, your degree of knowledge, experience, and focus is so deep that you can now see the whole picture with complete clarity, allowing you to perform your tasks with seemingly minimal effort. The skills, knowledge and movements have become hardwired into your brain and your muscles. Things begin to feel like second-nature.

There is now more intuition, you don't need to think so much about what you're doing. Seemingly somewhat effortless, your actions and behaviors engage your internal intuition and logic process. You improvise on the fly without consideration. It's as though you don't have to be conscious of your well-developed competence. You improvise. You just do it.

You truly now are a Creator. As you master your life, you will create beautiful things; bridges, flower gardens, artwork of all kinds, housing renovations, math equations, athletic displays, healthy kids, mechanical wonders, inspiring speeches, technological pathways, musical experiences or new ways to make love to your wife. You will begin to create your own realm of practice. You'll push into new opportunities. You'll begin to make stuff happen that you never knew you could do. You will begin to initiate unimagined possibilities and expand your life. This is mastery, the Creator.

One significant problem as we master anything is a concept called "Domain Dependent". This means that the domain that I have mastered works well only in one domain. For instance, a fish out of water does not look like the masterful swimmer he is. Or the world's best cellist has no competence in the octagon. These are extreme examples but do layout an aspect of how to master Masculinity.

Masculinity is domain independent. Masculinity is real, it is powerful, and it is influential across many domains, no matter if you are coaching little league baseball, running for political office or cooking dinner. But the pitfall would be to limit your vision and think it is only good at picking up women or in competitive sports. Or that it is inherently just a bad disturbance in the force. Masculinity is designed to cross many domains and remain significant wherever it goes.

⤳ Mastering your own life and your Masculinity prepares you well.

Mastery is a significant provider of power in every area of your life. If power is the ability to get something done, mastery seems to be the engine behind that. The more you pursue mastery, the more competence, freedom and influence you will have. Your capital, both social and financial will potentially increase. With more power, your ability to choose and create the life you want will increase. Your presence will become more noticed and influential everywhere you go. You will be more confident.

Until then, be ok with being a beginner. You are just starting.

Make it Happen; Master Your Masculinity

Now it is important to take the map that I have outlined as the skeleton and then begin to put the muscles on it. It is your task to take this information and give it life, to make it your own. Here are some steps to help you get this ball rolling in the right direction.

Assess where you are with Tension, Paradox and each Cornerstone, Currency, Benchmark, Muscle, Archetype and Distortion.

Cornerstones; Fortitude, Courage, Autonomy and Connection.

Currencies; Strength, Vulnerability, Freedom and Love.

Benchmarks; Power For, Solid Frame, Expansive, Passion

Muscles and TLA's; Provider (Build Your Capital), Protector (Build Your Power), Honor (Impeccable in Word and Deed), Integrity (Hold The Center), Explorer (Penetrate The Void), Initiator (Make Shit Happen), Thumos (Live Whole Hearted), Eros (Pursue Intimacy Passionately)

Achetypes; Warrior, King, Creator, Lover

Distortions; Power Over, Powerlessness, Unreliability, Spinelessness, Lack of Leadership, Passivity, Oblivious, the Domestic, Closed Heart, Impulsivity/Compulsivity and Abuse.

Determine which areas you want to develop and grow. You probably already know by what you just read what areas will need specific attention. Assessing will help you get an idea of what to prioritize first and what will be next. Or you could do a number of things at once, you make the plan.

Project manage this thing. Make it happen. According to Dr. Robert Glover, men are "Problem Solving Machines". So let's take that gift most of us have and create change in our lives! This book has outlined many concepts that can be built into the life of any man. Take the steps to build what you desire into your life.

Project management has a few steps, many of you do this every day with your work, just make it happen with yourself. First, Conceptualize a vision (what you want), then define your objectives (what it will look like) and then develop an intentional motivation (why you want to do this).

Next, develop a plan, outline the steps you'll take, consider potential obstacles and problems, and assess the resources you'll need. Problems may be if my wife doesn't want me to do this, or I don't have much money. Overcoming your obstacles is part of how Masculinity will grow in you. Resources may be books, podcasts, conferences, hiring a coach, attending a group, counseling, etc. It will take an investment, just like mastering anything.

Commit those resources to your project and begin to initiate the work implementing the steps you've outlined. As you continue through the project, assess your progress, continually re-assessing and making changes as needed to achieve your goals (what you want this to look like).

Begin the process of Mastering Your Masculinity.

Assess for yourself where your strengths, weaknesses and imbalances are. The idea is to build your masculine self into a balanced machine with all the aspects at play in your life. You will be naturally good at some of this and some will need to be built with intention.

Remember, this is about creating a good sense of how you want to build your own type and style of Masculinity. It is yours, make it what you want. Take the stuff I am outlining and build it how you want it to be. What I have outlined are significant parts of a masculine soul, how you develop it and balance it out is up to you with your personality and character.

There are Tension, Paradox, Cornerstones, Currencies, Benchmarks, Muscles, Archetypes and Distortions to assess. Take time to consider how well these are balanced into your life. Then make a plan to build the things you want to make happen first. This is a lifelong journey for each man, so make the plan for the long game. Make short-term plans and have an idea for the long-term goals as well.

It will be good just to write some stuff down about where you are. Have the beginner's mind and remember you are at the beginning stages of mastery. You are just an apprentice, this will take practice and repetition. First you just need to see where you are with each category, then make your plan. It will be very customized for you, because you are uniquely designed to carry this the way you are meant to. It can be very overwhelming but keep yourself steady and ready to build.

Get an idea of the masculine concepts you want to build in your life. There is no right or wrong, follow your intuition to grow and develop mastery of your Masculinity. Challenge yourself to do things that will push you into areas of discomfort and expose you to things you may have never considered.

My Vision; What do you now know about Masculinity and what do you want to build into your own life? What would you like to see in you?

My Objectives; Stay In Tension, Spend Currencies wisely, Build my Cornerstones, Build a Certain Benchmark, Muscle, TLA or Archetype.

My Motivation; I want to be strong, build a family, get better at my business, experience polarity with women, be influential, leave a legacy, etc.

My Plan; I am going to start with "A", "B" or "C". I will read "X". I will seek mentors. I will hire a coach. I will join a group of men, etc.

My Next Steps; The first thing I will do is_____. Then second, third, etc.

Potential Obstacles/Problems; My work schedule is too much. My finances are limited. My wife isn't ready for my changes. I have too high of a standard of living. I have too much debt. I don't believe in myself.

Needed Resources/Support; What do I need in place to get moving? Finances, relationships, time, energy, other men, etc. When will I start?

Assessment, Progress and Reassessment; See what you want to change.

Make Your Plan

List the top five things you want to build into your life first;

1)   2)   3)   4)   5)

What areas will be next;

1)   2)   3)   4)   5)

What are areas that will have to wait;

1)   2)   3)   4)   5)

Looking at the entire Map of Masculinity, which areas are you not excited about? And what areas are you chomping at the bit to build into your life?

THE SOLID MAN MAP OF MASCULINITY

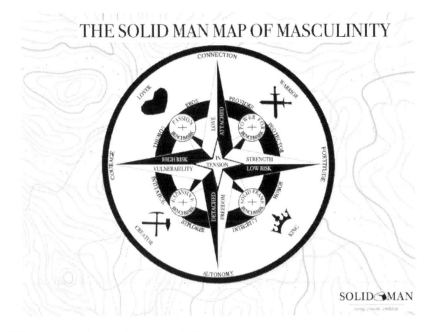

Which areas do you feel quite deficient in?

Which areas are you more proficient in?

What are areas you really want? Not excited about?

For each of those you listed to work on first, think of three things you could do to become more confident with that concept.

For instance, if you are not at all described as a man with a Thumos, you could; read Sam Keen's book, *Fire in the Belly*, read Paul Coughlin's book, *Unleashing Courageous Faith*, talk to anybody you know that has this kind of life, listen to podcasts about how men have built their passion for life, ask your friends what they think. This is going to take some research to get some great ideas. If you have a coach or mentor, they should have some ideas.

Do this the way you would do this. If you lean into the Solid Frame world and don't want to build a family, then don't, or do the opposite and build a family. If you have a more sensitive heart, do protection the way that kind of man does it; not so much with physical force, but vigilance and avoiding danger. Be a Warrior like you would do it, but be a Warrior. Be a King, Be a Creator. Be a Lover. Like you do it. Be intentional and make it happen..

This is all about defining and creating what/who you want to be as a man. It is the "be" not the "do" with your life. Remember that Masculinity is what you are, not what you do. As you seek to master this, make it your own. I have given you an outline of many characteristics, virtues and aspects of what a man is, now it is your turn to decide how it will look for you. Whatever that looks like, be that man with Passion and resolve.

Remember that you will start as an apprentice; gaining instruction and practicing basic fundamentals. This will take some time. This will be clumsy, so be patient and stay with it. This is where having other men along with you is essential, they will help you keep on the path.

Then when you begin to get this down, you'll move into the Creative-Active stage. In the trades world this is the Journeyman. You know what you're doing, you're good at what you do but it is not second nature yet. This is where you will plateau, which is very frustrating. Again, stay with it and be patient with yourself. Keep your men close by. They will help keep you going.

Eventually, you will begin to become a Master of your own self, to master your own Masculinity. You will be able to truly create the life that you want. You will make life that has all the things you want in it. You will be the man you have always wanted to be. That is your reward.

There are two books I would recommend on this topic, *Mastery*, by George Leonard and *Mastery* by Robert Greene. The authors come to the concept from different angles and each has a unique style of writing. Both books tell great stories about mastery and how to gain mastery in life.

⮡ Remember this: "Masculinity is a deep reality present within the core of every man. It is revealed in a drive to be a generous and powerful force for good, founded upon a solid internal integrity and identity, expressed through purposeful and creative movement into the world, and lived out with passion for life and relationship."

170

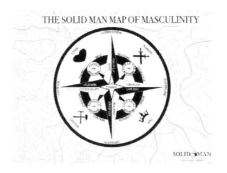

THE SOLID MAN MAP OF MASCULINITY

10 Conclusion

To master your Masculinity, you must know who you are. You must remember the deep truths that exist deep within you. You must awaken the internal realities of your masculine soul. You must find and join other men who are on this journey and men who have gone before you. You must find the true narrative of your life and throw out the BS that we have been taught about ourselves for the last half century or more.

> ➔ Look around you, which man do you want by your side in the zombie apocalypse? – Jack Donovan

The Map that I have presented here is a model, there are other models and ideas about Masculinity, so it doesn't matter what you do from here, except that you move forward with discovering who you really are as a man. From that, let your Internal Resources (Masculinity being a powerful resource) run your life. Not external narratives, what would make people happy with you or to live up to anyone else's expectations, do what you know is right.

Take all the information, ideas and concepts I have presented and begin to build your version of you, your version of your masculine self. All these concepts are essential to your masculine soul, how you play them out is up to you. You just have to make it so.

Remember who you are and be that man.

SOLID⬤MAN

---

strong · present · confident

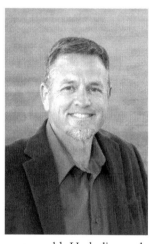

ABOUT THE AUTHOR

Ken Curry is a father, husband, mentor, friend and a Licensed Marriage and Family Therapist (LMFT) in Littleton, Colorado. His specialty is manhood, masculinity and relationships. He is continually exploring new avenues of strength, vitality and purpose for men.

Ken works from the premise that masculinity is good and that each man brings significance into our world. He believes that men have been designed to move with freedom, presence and strength. Along with individual and relationship counseling, Ken provides ongoing groups for men to build personal integrity in order to influence the world with intent and passion.

Ken has been developing the Solid Man Process so men can get their hearts back, develop their solid core, create freedom, grow healthy relationships, develop strength in their personal lives and overcome distracting issues like anger or porn. The Solid Man Process empowers men.

VISIT

⬤ SOLIDMAN.ORG

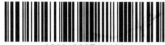

Made in the USA
Columbia, SC
30 June 2019